Colorectal Cancer

Colorectal Cancer

Edited by **Elaine Swan** BN(Hons), RGN, RM

Advanced Nurse Practitioner: Colorectal,
Manor Hospital, Walsall

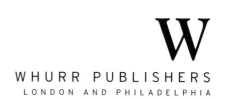

WHURR PUBLISHERS
LONDON AND PHILADELPHIA

© 2005 Whurr Publishers Ltd
First published 2005
by Whurr Publishers Ltd
19b Compton Terrace
London N1 2UN England and
325 Chestnut Street, Philadelphia PA 19106 USA

British Library Cataloguing in Publication Data

A catalogue record for this book
is available from the British Library.

ISBN 1 86156 334 5

Typeset by Adrian McLaughlin, a@microguides.net
Printed and bound in the UK by Athenæum Press Limited, Gateshead, Tyne & Wear

Contents

Contributors

Shelley Biddles, Colorectal Nurse Specialist, Queen's Medical Centre, Nottingham

Lucy Burgess, Nurse Specialist, Clinical Genetics Unit, Birmingham Woman's Hospital, Edgbaston, Birmingham

Helen Ferns, Colorectal Nurse Specialist, Colorectal Department, Clatterbridge Hospital, Bebington, Wirral

Yvette Perston, Colorectal Nurse Specialist, Llandough Hospital, Cardiff

Jonathan Stewart, Consultant Colorectal Surgeon, Walsall Manor Hospital, Honorary Senior Lecturer, Birmingham University

Elaine Swan, Advanced Nurse Practitioner – Colorectal, Manor Hospital, Walsall

Claire Taylor, Macmillan Colorectal CNS, Northwick Park and St Marks Hospital NHS, Harrow, Middlesex

Jane Winney, Colorectal Nurse Specialist, Stoma Care Department, Hereford County Hospital, Hereford

Preface

Colorectal Cancer covers all aspects of this subject that will benefit the nurse when caring for this group of patients.

Chapter 1 deals with the developing role of the colorectal nurse specialist to include professional accountability, managing change, assessing health care needs, specialist nurse/practitioner debate, specialist nursing practice and how this has evolved and changed over recent years. Chapter 2 explains the aetiology of colorectal cancer, how genes function, and the cancer/polyp multistep theory of colorectal carcinogenesis. Chapter 3 is concerned with epidemiology and genetics to include incidence of colorectal cancer, who is at increased risk, and the role of the clinical geneticist. Chapter 4 describes the diagnosis and investigations. Chapter 5 deals with treatment, surgery, mortality and follow-up. Chapter 6 is concerned with the consequences of rectal surgery, covering patient choice, informed consent, body image and sexuality. Chapter 7 relates to chemotherapy and radiotherapy and the oncology team. Finally, Chapter 8 is devoted to palliative care nursing and the support that can be offered to patients in the final stages of illness.

The aim of this book is to explain colorectal cancer to nurses in order to allow them to follow the patient's journey through diagnosis, treatment and aftercare. Bowels are a very sensitive area for many people to discuss, and the approach of the nurse within the multi-disciplinary team is all-important.

Acknowledgements

Many thanks to all those who contributed chapters for their hard work and enthusiasm. I am very grateful to friends and colleagues for their tireless support and encouragement. I should like to thank my family, daughters Amanda and Sarah and mom and dad, Babs and Ray and sister Debbi for their enduring love through difficult times.

> It does not matter how much or how little we achieve. If we don't jump for joy about it, we don't feel the emotional mileage.
>
> Astarius Reik-Om

Thank you to Sylvia, my secretary, without whose help I would not have been able to compile this book. Also many thanks to Maiya who gave me the strength and confidence to continue my work.

> Success is a journey, not a destination.
>
> Milton Erikson

Chapter 1

The role of the colorectal nurse specialist

Elaine Swan

The role of the clinical nurse specialist (CNS) remains an area of debate. Following the Briggs Report (Department of Health or DoH, 1972) the role of the CNS was introduced with the intention of improving the quality of patient care while also developing the career of senior nurses at existing ward sister level, to encourage them to stay within the clinical field of practice. The introduction of specialist nursing courses by the Joint Board of Clinical Studies, founded in 1970, provided the knowledge base and training for these nurses to develop. There are now a plethora of nurse specialists in all areas of practice with different titles, roles, levels of education and responsibility, and varying grades; this has led to much confusion within the profession and also for the general public.

McGee (1998) describes the specialist role as multidimensional; she says that there are a number of separate elements – care-giver, teacher, researcher, consultant, leader and manager – that can be identified; in reality they overlap and inform one another. She concludes that, although specialist practice should be regarded as a single entity, each practitioner has different strengths and develops the role in a way that suits both them and their employers. It is this freedom, she hypothesizes, that may be the essential ingredient in making such roles successful.

The role of the colorectal nurse specialist has developed and extended considerably. The UKCC document, *The Scope of Professional Practice* (UKCC, 1992), has allowed nurses to expand practice and take on new roles that may combine medical and nursing practice in order to promote a more holistic and effective approach to patient care. Fox (1995) suggested the notion of expansion of practice as acceptable when assisting in creating a comprehensive system of patient care. Collins (1989) noted that this should occur only where there are unmet needs of clients that are identified, or gaps in existing health care.

Professional accountability

As expansion of practice increases the workload, nurses must not compromise the service already established. Although Dyson (1990) felt that nurses would be able to undertake complex and challenging roles, it was highlighted by Autar (1996) that the nurse must be aware of not abdicating professional accountability by inappropriately delegating to others; nurses are legally accountable for their actions or omissions in care delivery (Nursing and Midwifery Council, 2002). A negligent practitioner may be subject to a professional conduct committee and/or local disciplinary proceedings. To cope with these developments and responsibilities in practice, the Nursing and Midwifery Council (NMC) emphasizes that all individual nurses, midwives and health visitors should carefully refer to their own personal experience, education and skill.

Hunt and Wainwright (1994) raise concerns of a professional and legal nature about the UKCC's (1992) document *The Scope of Professional Practice* and the possibilities of nurses developing their role and taking on activities that were previously the domain of other professionals. They highlight the lack of guidance concerning the competency levels of the practitioner and the expertise required to achieve this, leaving these decisions to be decided at an individual and hospital level. The law will judge anyone carrying out a medical procedure in comparison with a reasonable medical practitioner skilled in the procedure (*Bolam* v *Friern Hospital Management Committee*, 1957). By expanding roles, nurses must keep up to date with legal implications and the accountability that they must exercise. Tingle (1993) claimed that nurses must be aware of major areas of the law that relate to their sphere of professional practice, and that ignorance of the law is not acceptable.

For the nurse to develop successfully, a supportive management structure is required. The employer is legally responsible for its employees under vicarious liability. However, should the nurse undertake responsibilities outside the role, the nurse and not the employer is liable and can be sued for damages resulting from alleged negligence. Practitioners should, therefore, belong to an organization such as the Royal College of Nursing, or the Nursing branch of the Medical Defence Union, which have accepted the implications of the developing roles of nurses and can assist if problems arise and offer legal liability insurance to their members. Certainly, with increased autonomy, the nurse would assume greater legal responsibility, although Wright (1995) points out that the law is unclear and in need of clarification.

Managing change

Land et al. (1996) state that health care reform has emphasized that services should be flexible and ordered on the basis of the needs of individuals and client groups. This requires the efficient use of health care personnel and should also demonstrate clear and positive patient outcomes. Since the National Health Service Community Care Act 1990, which led to the separation between purchasing and providing health care, the responsibility of purchasers to assess health needs of their patients has been increasingly emphasized. Purchasers are evaluating the extent to which health care providers are meeting those needs and improving health.

Change is a necessary condition of survival, but we as individuals or organizations, with our differences, are a necessary ingredient in the change – the never-ending search for improvement. The challenge for the manager is to harness the energy and thrust of the differences so that the organization does not disintegrate but develops (Handy, 1993). Constant 'feedback' is necessary from patients, medical and nursing staff, and management. This can be gained through informal discussions, patient satisfaction surveys and independent performance review with management. Constant review of clinical practice within an annual report and within business plans allows for monitoring of progress, highlighting areas of concern and further developments planned, and also reporting on progress and achievements.

In the light of the White Paper, *Working for Patients* (DoH, 1989), the issue of auditing care has never been more important than it is today. The Government is firmly committed to efficiency, representing value for money; quality care can be achieved only through good management and regular audits of care. The purpose of quality assurance is to assure the consumer of nursing a specified degree of excellence through continuous measurement and evaluation (Schmadl, 1979). Auditing and evaluation of the service are essential. Auditing should be ongoing with the use of patient evaluation forms and the collection of statistical data on the efficiency, quality and effectiveness of the service.

The modernization of the NHS as set out in *The New NHS – Modern, Dependable* (DoH, 1997a) and *A First Class Service: Quality in the New NHS* (DoH, 1998) identify that providing effective nursing care to patients is essential. Nursing care should be evidence based, efficient and cost-effective. The introduction of clinical governance provides a framework for continuous improvement of the quality of services in the NHS and to safeguard high standards. There are seven pillars that need to be established within health care organizations in order to provide this environment:

- patient and public involvement
- clinical audit
- clinical risk management
- information
- staffing and staff management
- education, training and continuous personal and professional development
- research and clinical effectiveness.

Health care needs

The RCN document, *Public Health: Nursing rises to the challenge* (RCN, 1994), confirmed that health analysis is the first stage of taking public health perspectives forward into nursing practice. It stated that nurses are often closer to clients and their communities than other health workers, and so are uniquely placed to gain insight into local views and priorities. It suggested that nurses also have an important role as advocates for patients who may be unable to express their own views adequately from an informed perspective. Working with and alongside doctors, nurse specialists will be in an ideal position to act as advocates within the multidisciplinary team.

Demands for health care are ever increasing and are expected to rise further with an increasingly elderly population who are more dependent and have a greater tendency to ill-health. Interest in the environment, health issues and quality of service is growing. More people will take an active and responsible attitude to their own health, becoming less accepting of ill-health and more thoughtful and demanding consumers of health services (Heathrow Debate, 1993). In the past, health services have been very illness oriented; cure has traditionally been the province of medicine, care that of nurses. Increasingly nurses are becoming involved with those who are relatively healthy, aiming to raise the level of public health across society through health promotion, monitoring and support.

The Health of the Nation (DoH, 1992) strategy defined the aim of health education as being 'to ensure that individuals are able to exercise informed choice when selecting the lifestyle which they adopt'. Nursing is changing accordingly to meet these needs, making careful, thoughtful needs assessments using a methodical framework, but in a personal way offering information, advice and comfort to patients and carers, while acknowledging their individual identities and delivering effective care. Evaluation, effectiveness and value for money are key issues, and nurses and other health care professionals are much more accountable for the service they provide.

Nurse practitioner

With the reduction of junior doctors' hours in 1991, the NHS Management Executive suggested that nurses could be trained to take on work that was previously carried out by junior doctors. It is interesting to note that Nemes (1994) described the nurse practitioner role as not a doctor's substitute but a role that strengthens and promotes a multidisciplinary approach to patient care. Nevertheless, this change to junior doctors' hours has provided a focus for change. A partnership approach between medical and nursing staff would establish teamwork rather than a hierarchical structure in a multidisciplinary team, but Wright (1995) states that nurses should not be protective towards their practice, or argue about professional boundaries, because this indicates a power struggle rather than acting in the best interest of the patient. Marsden (1995) stresses the importance of communication with medical colleagues in order to assess their response, gain their support and identify areas where a nurse practitioner role would be effective, and what he or she would be able to do.

The British Society of Gastroenterology's Working Party (1995) supported the proposition that suitably trained and supervised nurses should carry out certain types of diagnostic endoscopy, i.e. flexible sigmoidoscopy. Also stressed in this document is that medico-legally a nurse may perform an endoscopy provided that she or he has received the appropriate training, has the support of the health authority/trust and is adequately supervised by the responsible consultant. There are several established posts in the USA where nurses perform screening flexible sigmoidoscopy and this has demonstrated that nurses can develop practical skills in medical procedures comparable to those of their medical colleagues (Disario and Sanowski, 1993; Maule, 1994). There are now many nurses in the UK who perform endoscopies and have done so for several years. They have expanded their roles to include therapeutics, managing their own lists and running services. The impetus for the training and recruitment of nurse endoscopists has been the 2-week waiting time rule for suspected cancer: in 2000, in response to long waiting lists, the Government pledged that a specialist would see patients with suspected cancer within two weeks of referral by their GP.

The definition of a specialist was open to interpretation, which meant that they could be seen by a nurse specialist or a doctor. Some nurses have set up open-access endoscopy clinics for these urgent cases and refer patients if they need further investigations. Other specialist nurses have set up similar clinics for non-urgent cases to relieve the burden on the consultant colorectal clinics by dealing with the more minor referrals, enabling them to see cancer cases more quickly.

Improving patient care

There is a growing need for colorectal nurse specialists to provide continuity of care in the patient's pathway from diagnosis to surgical, adjuvant and palliative treatments, and to liaise among the patient, primary care doctor and the hospital services (Association of Coloproctology of Great Britain and Ireland or ACPGB&I, 2001). The Calman Report (Calman and Hine, 1995), 'A policy framework for commissioning cancer services', advised a multidisciplinary team working approach to patient and carers as being central to the service. Current Government policy emphasizes the need for improved communication with patients and their families and good continuity of care, and they recognize the role that nurses have in improving care (DoH, 2000a).

The publication of *Improving Outcomes in Colorectal Cancer: The manual* (DoH, 1997b) provides good evidence that specialist nurses working as part of a multidisciplinary palliative care team can reduce patients' distress, improve pain control, and increase satisfaction and information flow to patients. They recommended that there were a number of operational possibilities for fulfilling this nurse specialist role and that this nurse should be available to all colorectal cancer patients. The Commission for Health Improvement (CHI, 2001) reviewed cancer services throughout the UK; they reported that some progress had been made but there was scope for improving interprofessional communication.

The NHS Plan: A plan for investment, a plan for reform (DoH, 2000b, 2000c) – for improving nurses' role and numbers – sets out the requirement that NHS employers empower appropriately qualified nurses, midwives and therapists to undertake a wider range of clinical tasks, including the right to make referrals, admit and discharge patients, order investigations and diagnostic tests, run clinics and prescribe drugs.

Specialist nursing practice

The role of the colorectal nurse specialist encompasses many aspects, i.e. clinical, teaching, research and management. Specialist nursing practice was defined by the UKCC (1994) in its document of standards for post-registration education and practice as:

> practice for which the nurse is required to possess additional knowledge and skill in order to exercise a higher level of clinical judgement and discretion in clinical care and to provide expert clinical care and leadership, teaching and supporting others.

The specialist nurse/practitioner is expected to be at first-degree level. The UKCC did not give a definition of 'an advanced nursing practitioner'. Castledine (1994) comments that this person will be expected to have higher knowledge and skills than a specialist nursing practitioner. Such an individual should be able to provide expert clinical care, clinical leadership, management, teaching, supervision and support. The UKCC document *Prep and You* (1993) acknowledges that practitioners are acquiring advanced skills and undertaking studies that are likely to be at Masters and PhD level. The recording of such qualifications may be considered in due course. The nurse practitioners' role developed in the USA in the mid-1960s as a response to a shortage of doctors available to provide primary care. The initiative developed and expanded and led to a number of education programmes, mainly at Masters level.

There is some confusion in the UK surrounding the term 'nurse practitioner' and its relationship to other nursing titles such as clinical nurse specialist, advanced practitioner, nurse clinical, etc.; the debate within the profession has yet to come to a conclusion about definition and educational level requirements. Castledine (1993) suggests that the primary activities of nurse practitioners include screening, physical and psychosocial assessment, health promotion, health education, patient teaching, medical techniques, drug prescribing, medical and diagnostic testing, certification of inevitable death, counselling and co-ordination of care.

In the 'Scope' document, the UKCC (1992) rejects the notion of 'role extension' which limited the parameters of practice. It was envisaged that, through role expansion, professional discretion can be enhanced. Nurses can take their own initiative, do their own thinking and make their own decisions based on their own experience and education, to improve practice for the benefit of patients and clients. Role expansion should progress in recognition of the health care needs of society/communities, and this purposeful progression will lead to the acceptance of new responsibilities that are appropriate to this end (Hunt and Wainwright, 1994).

Over 34 000 new cases of bowel cancer are diagnosed in the UK each year. Colorectal cancer is the third most common cause of cancer death, accounting for one in eight of all cancers (Cancer Research Campaign, 2001). More resources are being directed to cancer services by the Government; through multidisciplinary team management, colorectal cancer patients will benefit.

Greater public awareness of the symptoms of bowel disorders and increased public demand for quicker, more responsive services and information has increased pressure on health service professionals (ACPGB&I, 2001). Colorectal cancer follow-up is one area of care that has been identified to be developed by colorectal nurse specialists; consultant staff will not be able to cope with the total workload of patients with colorectal disease (ACPGB&I, 2001) in this rapidly expanding area. An expansion of practice increases the workload; the CNS must not compromise the already established service, and appropriate clerical and nursing personnel must be agreed and in place before this can be undertaken. For the nurse to develop successfully, a supportive management structure is required. By expanding roles, nurses must keep up to date with legal implications and the accountability that they must exercise.

The colorectal nurse practitioner role has developed to involve the setting up and running of nurse-led services in early cancer detection, cancer follow-up clinics, health promotion and screening, including sigmoidoscopy, anorectal physiology investigations and faecal continence management. The details of the role need to be discussed with the multidisciplinary team members involved, and protocols and guidelines developed for certain procedures to be undertaken by the nurse practitioner. Role development expansion must take place alongside protocols and clear guidelines for practice devised within the parameters of *The Scope of Practice* (UKCC, 1992) and *The Code of Professional Conduct* (NMC, 2002) to ensure that the practitioner practises to her or his limitations, always retaining the patient as the focus of all care. The educational needs of the practitioner must be identified and addressed and also the ongoing supervision of practice with an identified clinical supervisor. Koch et al. (1992) reported that, where nurse practitioner roles had been evaluated, they appeared to have a positive effect on patient outcomes.

The report of the RCN/Coloplast Competencies Project published in 2002 outlines the roles and boundaries of nurses caring for people with colorectal problems and defines the competencies required for those working in this field. In line with clinical governance (DoH, 1998), those nurses in specialist roles need to be able to demonstrate minimum levels of competence in order to ensure that high-quality nursing care is achieved. Colorectal nurse specialists need additional knowledge and skills in order to deliver innovative, effective and evidence-based care (RCN, 2002). This document was developed from the views and expertise of over 50 per cent of the specialists to whom the document relates, and also includes the views of patients. Within the document, the expert competencies common to all areas of practice are described under these headings:

- advocacy
- consultancy
- initiation of new work
- research

- work beyond the organization
- team management.

An individual practitioner can use her or his own specialist knowledge to apply these competencies to areas of expert practice. This report provides a comprehensive picture of the competencies needed for this area of practice, and an invaluable tool that can be used for:

- articulating the value of nurses in this area of practice
- clarifying roles and boundaries of practice
- matching service needs to current education/professional development provision
- formulating job descriptions
- preparing person specifications
- selection and recruitment
- career progression
- continuing professional development
- contributing to the competency/expert practice debate.

The NMC has recently revised the professional nursing register. Since November 2003 the register has been divided into three sections: nursing, midwifery and specialist community public health nursing. This will protect, in law, the titles for specialist roles; nurses will not be able to use the title unless appropriately qualified to do so and unless they have been assessed and recorded as such by the NMC.

Porrett (1996) describes the attitude of society with regard to elimination, where bowels are a taboo subject and there is a perceived stigma attached to these 'below the waist' conditions; this has presumably affected the provision of colorectal services. Much can be achieved through health education to change attitudes, raise public awareness and empower people to take responsibility for their own health. Attending the outpatient department clinic will enable the nurse practitioner to offer more support, information and advice to patients. Pearson (1989) suggested that patients need nurses to humanize the system for them and help them to overcome any sense of abandonment in the health service. Nurses become experts in coaching a patient through an illness; they take what is foreign and fearful to the patient and make it familiar and less frightening (Benner, 1984).

Egan (1982) described his model of counselling as a problem management model, applicable to any context in which people need help. It is, therefore, not limited to the psychological realm, but can easily encompass general health care. The approach is essentially a very good framework for helping, or more accurately for helping people help themselves. This model has been adapted and used to improve counselling skills with patients. Public awareness of bowel disease can be raised by organizing open days, and developing educational information, i.e. posters and leaflets for displays. More information should empower people to seek early advice from their doctor if they can overcome stigma and embarrassment surrounding this subject. The colorectal nurse specialist/practitioner will need to act as a resource person to the multidisciplinary team and organize educational programmes in order to update health-care staff on the latest developments within colorectal disease management. This strategy should include community health care staff, because they are the first-line personnel more likely to have initial contact with patients and, in terms of early cancer detection, are of the utmost importance.

Colorectal nurse specialists are an example of patient-based expert practitioners (UKCC, 1994) who are ideally suited and located to develop and enhance nursing services in the area of colorectal disease. It holds great challenges and opportunities for the nurse wishing to expand knowledge and skills. The current climate allows nurses to be proactive and choose to develop rather than waiting for things to happen.

If nurses do not take on new roles, others will, which may militate against holistic patient care (Autar, 1996). Within the new proposed health care reforms, nurses are in a good position to respond and embrace these specialist roles; they provide for professional growth and change.

Table of cases

Bolam v Friern Hospital Management Committee [1957] All ELR 2, 118.

References

Association of Coloproctology of Great Britain and Ireland (2001) Resources for Coloproctology. London: Association of Coloproctology of Great Britain and Ireland.

Autar R (1996) Role of the nurse teacher in advanced nursing practice. British Journal of Nursing 5: 298-301.

Benner P (1984) from Novice to Expert: Excellence and power in clinical nursing practice. Menlo Park, Calif: Addison-Wesley.

Breeze J (1995) Stoma care: is there room to extend our practice? British Journal of Nursing 4: 1001-1005.

British Society of Gastroenterology (1995) The Nurse Endoscopist – Report of the Working Party of the British Society of Gastroenterology. London: BSG.

Calman K, Hine D (1995) Expert Advisory Group on Cancer. A Policy Framework for Commissioning Cancer Services London: Department of Health and Welsh Office.

Cancer Research Campaign (2001) Facts about Cancer. London: CRC (www.crc.org.uk).

Castledine G (1993) Nurse Practitioner title: ambiguous and misleading. British Journal of Nursing 2: 734-735.

Castledine G (1994) Advanced and specialist nursing and the scope of practice. In: Hunt G, Wainwright P (eds), Expanding the Role of the Nurse. London: Blackwell Science Ltd.

Collins HL (1989) Find a need and meet it. Registered Nurse 52(10): 61-62 cited by Breeze (1995).

Commission for Health Improvement (2001) National Service Frameworks Assessments No. 1. NHS Cancer Care in England and Wales. London: CHI.

Department of Health (1972) Briggs Report. London: HMSO.

Department of Health (1989) Working for Patients. London: DoH.

Department of Health (1992) The Health of the Nation. London: HMSO.

Department of Health (1997a) The New NHS - Modern, Dependable. London: DoH

Department of Health (1997b) Improving Outcomes in Colorectal Cancer: The manual. London: DoH.

Department of Health (1998) A First Class Service: Quality in the new NHS. London: DoH.

Department of Health (2000a) The NHS National Cancer Plan. London: HMSO.

Department of Health (2000b) The Nursing Contribution to Cancer Care - A strategic programme of action in support of the national cancer programme. London: HMSO.

Department of Health (2000c) The NHS Plan - A plan for investment, a plan for reform. London: HMSO.

Disario JA, Sanowski RA (1993) Sigmoidoscopy training for nurses and resident physicians. Gastrointestinal Endoscopy 39: 29-32.

Dyson R (1990) Changing Labour Utilisation in NHS Trusts. University of Keele.

Egan G (1982) The Skilled Helper. Monterey, Calif: Brooks/Cole.

Fox P (1995) nursing developments: trust nurses' views. Nursing Standard 4: 938-939.

Handy C (1993) Understanding Organisations, 4th edn. London: Penguin Books Ltd.

Heathrow Debate (1993) Nursing Strategy Workshop 'Health and Social Care 2010 - shaping the future'. Chief Nursing Officers, England, Wales, Scotland and Northern Ireland.

Hunt G, Wainwright P (eds) (1994) Expanding the Role of the Nurse: The scope of professional practice. London: Blackwell Science Ltd.

Koch L et al. (1992) The first 20 years of nurse practitioner literature. Nurse Practitioner 17 (2): 62-71: cited by Porrett (1996).

Land L, Mhaolrunaigh SN, Castledine G (1996) Extent and effectiveness of the Scope of Professional Practice. Nursing Times 92(35): 32-35.

McGee P (1998) Specialist practice in the UK. In: Castledine G, McGee P (eds), Advanced and Specialist Nursing Practice. London: Blackwell Science.

Marsden J (1995) Setting up nurse practitioner roles: issues in practice. British Journal of Nursing 4: 948-952.

Maule WF (1994) screening for colorectal cancer by nurse endoscopists. New England Journal of Medicine 330: 183-187.

Nursing and Midwifery Council (2002) The Code of Professional Conduct. London: NMC.

Nemes J (1994) Nurse practitioner in acute care units. Nursing Standard 9(8): 37-39.

Pearson A (1989) Trends in Clinical Nursing. Primary nursing. London: Croom Helm.

Porrett T (1996) Extending the role of the stoma care nurse. Nursing Standard 10(27): 33-35.

Royal College of Nursing (1994) Public Health: Nursing rises to the challenge. London: RCN.

Royal College of Nursing (2002) Competencies in Nursing. Caring for people with colorectal problems. The RCN/Coloplast Competencies Report. London: RCN.

Schmadl JC (1979) Quality assurance: Examination of the concept. Nursing Outlook 27: 462-465.

Tingle JH (1993) The extended role of the nurse, legal implications. Care of the Critically Ill 9(1): 30.

United Kingdom Central Council of Nursing and Midwifery (1992) The Scope of Professional Practice. London: UKCC.

United Kingdom Central Council of Nursing and Midwifery (1993) Prep and You. London: UKCC.

United Kingdom Central Council of Nursing and Midwifery (1994) The Future of Professional Practice – The Council's standard for education and practice following registration, London: UKCC.

Winawer SJ, Miller DG, Sherlock P (1984) Risk and screening for colorectal cancer. Advances in Internal Medicine 30: 471–496.

Wright S (1995) The role of the nurse: extended or expanded. Nursing Standard 9(33): 25–29.

Chapter 2

Aetiology of colon and rectal cancer

Jonathan Stewart

Genes and colorectal cancer

Colon and rectal cancers develop by the accumulation of changes that occur in certain genes within the cells of the mucosal lining of the bowel (Fearon and Vogelstein, 1990). The genes that are mainly affected appear to have important roles in the control of the cell cycle, differentiation, contact inhibition, angiogenesis and many other regulatory mechanisms of cellular growth. The alterations that occur in these genes can arise as a result of exposure to carcinogens (e.g. chemicals, dietary, viral or irradiation), spontaneous sporadic mutation, or an inherited gene defect (Hall, 1998a). There is also some evidence that environmental factors such as diet may affect certain gene mechanisms. The changes may also arise on the background of chronic diseases such as ulcerative colitis.

There would appear to be two molecular pathways that may result in the development of colorectal cancers. The first pathway to be described was the now-classic adenomatous polyp–cancer sequence or multistep mutation. This theory states that there is a progressive mutation of oncogenes and loss of the function of tumour suppressor genes (Bishop, 1985). By employing mathematical models that study tumour growth there is now evidence that several genetic events have to occur to develop an invasive colon tumour. The gradual accumulation of these genetic events will usually require several years (often 10–20) and is therefore consistent with the epidemiological data regarding the polyp–cancer sequence (Nordling, 1953; Hall, 1998b).

The second, more recently described, is the replication error (RER) or microsatellite instability (MIS) pathway. Genes responsible for DNA-mismatch repair mediate this pathway. Our knowledge remains incomplete, but it would appear that several classes of genes are involved in the transformation of normal colonic mucosa to malignant. They include:

- oncogenes
- tumour suppressor genes
- DNA-repair genes.

The purpose of this chapter is to describe some of the molecular and biological principles that are involved in the aetiology of colorectal cancer.

In 1866 Paul Broca, while mapping his wife's family tree, noted a hereditary predisposition to develop cancers. His observations were largely ignored until 1914, when Boveri proposed that changes in chromosomes were related to malignancy. It is now accepted that genetic alterations in the normal genome can result in the formation of tumours.

The identification of a genetic aetiology for cancer came in 1960, with the description of a specific acquired abnormality, the Philadelphia (Ph') chromosome in chronic myeloid leukaemia (Nowell, 1960). This chromosomal abnormality was termed a 'translocation' (Klein, 1981). A portion of genetic material was moved from one chromosome to another, which resulted in an abnormal expression of the genetic information. These and other observations led to the concept that certain genes regulated growth and cell division and they could be 'activated' in an abnormal manner if they were translocated to another area on a chromosome that contained a 'promoter' area.

In 1910, Peyton Rous demonstrated that cell-free extracts of chicken sarcomas could induce tumours when injected into host animals (Rous, 1911). This was a demonstration that a type of virus termed a 'retrovirus' could induce tumours (Bishop, 1987). Since those early experiments a group of genes originally found attached to certain retroviruses has now been identified. These genes have been termed 'oncogenes' (Vogelstein et al., 1988; Aaltonen et al., 1993; Kinzler and Vogelstein, 1998).

Genetic instability is the basis for the development of colorectal cancer. This process may occur in two broad and possibly overlapping ways. The instability may affect the whole chromosome or short segments of repetitive DNA termed 'microsatellites' (Senba et al., 1998).

Microsatellite instability and DNA-repair genes

Microsatellites are unique repeated segments of DNA. These base segments usually consist of cytosine (C) and adenine (A) nucleotides, or dinucleotides (CA repeats). These segments are found scattered throughout the genome. Their exact function remains unknown.

In tumours it has been found that these repeated segments are often altered. Typically new alleles may appear, indicating a failure of DNA replication. This failure of DNA replication was termed 'microsatellite instability' or MSI (Aaltonen et al., 1993). The failure of the normal replication is thought to result from loss of normal function in the DNA polymerase during replication. The cell subsequently fails to recognize the mismatch. It was the detection of MSI in hereditary non-polyposis coli (HNPC) cancers that led to the discovery of DNA-mismatch repair (MMR) genes.

Studies have suggested that DNA MMR gene deficiency (caused by mutation of *hMSH2*, *hMLH1*, *hPMS1* or *hPMS2* genes) contributes to the development of HPNC (Lynch syndrome). Most tumours in these patients display MSI. DNA-repair genes are thought to play a part in tumour development by the loss of protein function. After such a loss certain tumour suppressor genes and oncogenes may undergo mutation with progression to neoplastic change.

The failure of the cell to recognize and repair the mismatch or defect probably promotes carcinogenesis through the loss of a caretaker function in certain genes. The loss of such a self-regulatory mechanism may result in the accumulation of other genetic errors or mutations (Thibodeau et al., 1998). The areas of DNA that appear to be particularly prone to the loss of MMR are segments of DNA that contain repeated short segments. The progressive accumulation of defects occurs in the cancer cells (Ionov et al., 1993).

Studies have demonstrated that approximately 15 per cent of sporadic colorectal cancers contain MSI. It would appear, therefore, that there are other mechanisms for the development of MSI (Cairns, 1981).

Oncogenes

Oncogenes were originally detected in certain tumour-forming viruses (Weiss, 1982). Oncogenes are in fact normal genes but when they become inappropriately activated or expressed they may result in the development of disease (Duesberg, 1983). The products of the oncogenes tend to have vital roles in the control of the cell cycle, growth and differentiation (Bishop, 1981). The activation or expression in an abnormal manner of these genes, and hence in their protein products, can result in a neoplastic transformation. The loss of normal growth control, contact inhibition and other functions gives the cell the ability to invade surrounding tissues and even metastasis (Hamlyn, 1984): the cell has become malignant (Roberts and Pembrey, 1985). A number of oncogenes have been identified and are thought to play a role in the development of colorectal cancers.

These, then, are some of the building blocks involved in the development of neoplasia (Marshall, 1984). The classic polyp–cancer sequence and the role of MSI theories probably have areas of overlap depending on a given situation. There still remain significant gaps in our knowledge about the pathways and specific triggers that initiate the process.

How do genes function?

Cellular DNA is composed of 22 pairs of autosomal chromosomes and one pair of sex chromosomes (XX or XY). The 22 pairs of chromosomes contain the 100 000 or so genes that make up the human genome. Two copies, termed 'alleles', one inherited from each parent, represent each gene. Each allele of a gene is located at a specific place or locus on the paternal and maternal strands of DNA. There may be some subtle differences between each allele, which are termed 'polymorphisms'. These polymorphisms may have little or no effect on the gene product. Some changes, however, may cause such a dramatic change in the gene product that the way in which the gene functions may be altered. Some of these changes may predispose to, or result in, the development of diseases. Such a change is termed a 'mutation' (Knudson, 1985).

Mutations or the inappropriate activation of genes can occur in a variety of ways (Hansen and Cavenee, 1987), including the following:

- infection by certain types of viruses
- chromosomal translocations
- gene amplification
- point mutations.

Gene products are the proteins encoded by the gene DNA sequences. DNA consists of a double-stranded polymer, the monomeric units of which are the nucleotide bases, adenosine (A), guanosine (G), thymidine (T) and cytosine (C). The ability of a particular region of the DNA strand to code for a particular protein is determined by the sequence of the four bases along that region of the chain. Different combinations of the bases code for different amino acids, and thus for the proteins that they make up. The sequences are decoded by the cell's protein synthesis machinery in codons or groups of three bases (ATG, GAC, TAG, GAC).

A change in the structure or order of the codons may alter the gene product to such an extent that the function of a particular protein may be altered or lost. If the protein plays an important role in the regulation of cell structure or growth the cell will become abnormal. If the cell obtains a growth advantage it may become malignant. In certain situations the alteration of one matched copy is sufficient to cause a phenotypic change. This is termed a 'dominant' condition; examples of such diseases include polycystic kidney and familial adenomatous polyposis (FAP). If changes in both alleles are required to alter the function, the condition is termed 'recessive' (e.g. cystic fibrosis).

Tumour suppressor genes

Oncogenes often tend to function in a dominant fashion. There is, however, another class of genes that function in a recessive manner. These are termed 'tumour suppressor genes' (De Mars, 1969; Knudson, 1971).

Tumour suppressor genes are a class of genes with normal function that appear to be related to the control or suppression of cell proliferation. The inactivation of these genes results in the loss of normal cell growth control. It has been proposed that a mutation of one copy of this type of gene was inherited in such conditions as FAP and that neoplasms resulted from the subsequent somatic mutation of the normal allele (Markowitz et al., 1995). It was later proposed that the same germline genes would be altered somatically in the development of both the familial and the non-familial type of bowel cancers (Parsons et al., 1995).

The inactivation of tumour suppressor genes during the development of tumours is often associated with the loss of some of the tumour suppressor DNA. This loss may be detected using sophisticated molecular biological techniques. One such technique is to detect the loss of restriction fragment length polymorphism alleles in the tumour DNA which are present in normal DNA from the same person. The loss of such constitutional heterozygosity in tumours may be employed to detect the sites of tumour suppressor genes.

An example of a tumour suppressor gene is the R_{II} gene. This gene codes for the transforming growth factor-β_2 (TGF-β_2) receptor (Kingsley, 1994). This gene is an inhibitor of cell growth in the bowel and is also involved in the induction of apoptosis (programmed cell death). Programmed cell death was discovered in 1972 (Kerr, Wyllie and Currie, 1972). Cancers can develop when mutations affect the control mechanisms of apoptosis and cell survival. There is now known to be a 'family' of such proteins that appear to have a variety of functions to do with the control of cell growth (Massague, 1990). These proteins can be divided into three broad subclasses: TGF-β, activins and decapentaplegic protein (DPP). The gene has a special area within its coding region (termed 'A10'), which seems to make it susceptible to mutations in MMR-deficient cells. In tumours with MSI, 80–90 per cent appear to have a mutated R_{II} poly(A) region (Souza et al., 1996).

The insulin-like growth factor II receptor (IGF-IIR) is mutated in a similar way. This mutation appears less commonly than the R_{II} mutation and, interestingly, not in tumours in which the R_{II} mutation has occurred (Nowell, 1976). It would appear, therefore, that one or probably more of these types of tumour suppressor genes are necessary for tumours with MSI to develop. These might include other types of MMR genes or hypomethylation of the MMR genes, leading to altered function (Bodmer, Bishop and Karran, 1994).

DNA methylation

DNA methylation plays a complex role in the development of tumours. Hypomethylation is associated with increase in gene expression and may play a role in the activation of oncogenes such as *k-ras*. Similarly, DNA hypermethylation can coexist with hypomethylation in different areas of the genome in a variety of tumours.

The multistep, polyp-cancer theory of colorectal carcinogenesis

Based on the available epidemiological and molecular evidence, it is now apparent that a multistep pathway is involved in the development of colorectal cancers. In 1976 Nowell proposed the clonal theory of carcinogenesis (Vogelstein et al., 1988). Colorectal cancers arise from a single cell that develops by clonal expansion. Genetic events gradually accumulate in clones of cells. These events may be acquired by mutations or be inherited. Some changes would be deleterious to the cell, others would give it a growth advantage. Those cells that developed a growth advantage would gradually produce a subclone of cells that would continue to grow. Gradually further clones would develop and, with successive mutations accumulating within the cells, a polyp; then, gradually with time and further gene changes, a malignant cancer would develop (Groden et al., 1991). This theory explained the time lag from patients developing polyps and subsequently tumours in later life. Histological analysis of tumours helps to confirm the theory because analysis often reveals the presence of adenomatous tissue adjacent to the tumour. The tumour has arisen as a clone from the polyp cells.

In 1988 Vogelstein et al. reasoned that the pattern of change that occurred in certain genes in colorectal cancers might be reflected in the different stages of development of tumours during the transition from normal mucosa to polyp and subsequent cancer (Nakamura, 1995). The numbers of altered genes that occur in either oncogenes or tumour suppressor genes appear to be more critical than the exact order in which they occur. There are several genes that have been identified as playing a role in this multistep pathway (Figure 2.1).

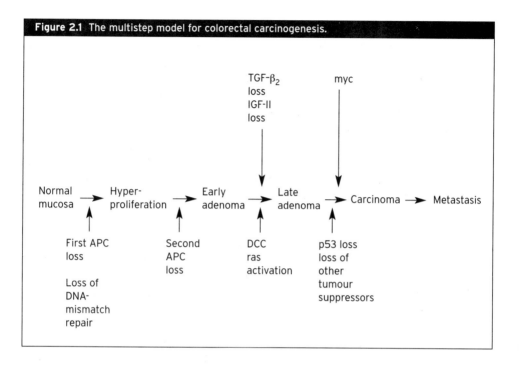

Figure 2.1 The multistep model for colorectal carcinogenesis.

The *APC* gene

The investigation for the genetic cause of FAP resulted in the discovery of the adenomatous polyposis gene (*APC*). Further research has led to the identification that the *APC* gene is one of the most important targets in the development of colorectal cancers. The *APC* gene is expressed in most tissues and is composed of 19 exons, 16 of which are alternatively expressed. (The significance of these multiple transcripts is not known.) The gene encodes for a protein composed of 2843 amino acids.

The *APC* gene occurs on chromosome 5q21 (Kinzler et al., 1991). The deletion of the 5q area (the site of the gene) is found in over 30 per cent of colorectal adenomatous polyps, but it is not more common in sporadic colorectal cancers. Experiments have demonstrated that the loss of chromosome 5 allele occurs in both sporadic and FAP cancers and adenomatous polyps, but not in FAP polyps (Kinzler and Vogelstein, 1996). The available evidence indicates that the *APC* gene functions as a tumour suppressor gene.

The *APC* gene has been termed a 'gatekeeper gene'. It would appear that it is probably involved in the initiation of adenomatous polyps (Northover and Murday, 1989). In the development of sporadic polyps, both copies of the *APC* gene must probably be inactive. This permits the initiating trigger for the development of a polyp. As the function of the *APC* gene is lost, a polyp with the potential for malignant transformation (depending on which other gene mechanisms are affected) forms.

From the studies to date it would appear that the *APC* gene aids in the control of cell growth by several mechanisms. These include regulation of cell adhesion, processing of signalling pathways, maintaining the cytoskeleton, and cell cycle progression and apoptosis (Spirio et al., 1993; Morin, Vogelstein and Kinzler, 1996). The loss or inactivation of the *APC* gene results in the disruption of the normal balance between cell division and death. The result is disordered growth.

Familial adenomatous polyposis

There are several rare inherited syndromes that predispose to the development of colorectal cancers. One of the best studied is familial adenomatous polyposis or FAP. Studies of this disease have resulted in insights into the development of non-inherited colorectal cancers. FAP is an autosomal dominant condition in which multiple polyps develop throughout the colon and rectum. The patients will usually develop a colorectal cancer in their 20s to 40s unless they undergo a prophylactic panproctocolectomy either with a Pouch anal reconstruction or a permanent ileostomy. The patients are also at a greater risk of developing other malignancies. In addition, duodenal polyps are discovered in a similar manner in these patients. Desmoid tumours develop in 4 per cent of FAP patients.

Investigations have revealed that there appear to be specific sites of *APC* gene mutation that are related to specific phenotypes of familial adenomatosis coli. Patients with profuse polyposis develop more than 5000 adenomas. There is an attenuated form that is usually associated with an older age and lower number of polyps (Bussey, 1975; Lynch et al., 1995).

In patients with FAP, a germline mutation of the *APC* gene has taken place. This is followed by somatic mutation or deletion of the remaining allele in colon cancer cells. FAP is associated with almost complete penetrance and has an estimated frequency of 1 in 10 000. About 20 per cent of patients with FAP have no family history of their disease. It is thought that they carry spontaneous new mutations of the *APC* gene.

In a distinct phenotype variant of FAP, colorectal polyps are associated with epidermoid cysts, fibromas and osteomas. This syndrome is termed 'Gardner's syndrome' (Gardner and Richards, 1953). Patients with Turcot's syndrome (colorectal cancers and medulloblastomas) also have a variant of FAP and carry germline *APC* mutations (Hamilton et al., 1995).

Several other genes have now been demonstrated to play a role in the development of colorectal cancers (Table 2.1).

Table 2.1 Some genes involved in the development of colorectal cancers

Gene	Chromosomal site	Syndrome	Protein
APC	5q21	FAP	Cell adhesion, control c-myc, apoptosis
hMSH2	2p16	HNPCC	DNA-mismatch repair
HMLH1	3p21	HNPCC	DNA-mismatch repair
p53	17p13	Tumour suppressor repair DNA damage, apoptosis	Cell cycle control,
DCC	18q21	Tumour suppressor	Cell adhesion
MCC	5q21	Tumour suppressor	Not known
K-ras	12p	Oncogene	GTP binding
c-myc	8q24	Oncogene	DNA synthesis
R11		Tumour suppressor	TGF-β_2 receptor gene
IGF-IIR	6q26	Tumour suppressor	Activation of TGF-β

FAP, familial adenomatous polyposis; HNPCC, hereditary non-polyposis coli cancer; TGF, transforming growth factor.

The *MCC* gene

The *MCC* (mutated in colorectal cancer) gene is located on chromosome 5q21, close to the FAP gene. The gene codes for a protein of 829 amino acids, which is similar in structure to that of the *APC* gene product. It is possible that they interact in some way, although at present their exact function remains unknown.

The *p53* gene

Protein p53 is produced by a gene located on the short arm of chromosome 17 (17p13), and this gene codes for a 53-kDa nuclear phosphoprotein that contains 393 amino acids. It appears to act as a tumour suppressor-type gene. Not only do a high proportion (70 per cent) of colorectal cancers demonstrate loss of the allele responsible for the production of the oncoprotein *p53*, but also the abnormality is detected in nearly half of all tumours (Harris and Hollstein, 1993). Point mutations in *p53* have been detected in regions of the gene in colorectal cancers but only rarely in adenomatous polyps. The inactivation of *p53* appears to be associated with the transition mechanism from a benign to a malignant polyp. In the development of colorectal neoplasms, *p53* function can be lost by a combination of chromosomal mutation and deletion by the loss of heterozygosity. The *p53* can also lose its function when only one allele is mutated because the mutant *p53* can bind to the wild-type *p53* inactivating it (a dominant negative effect). The fact that *p53* seems to play a central pivotal role in maintaining the stability of DNA has earned it the title of 'guardian of the genome' (Kern et al., 1992).

The *p53* gene seems to possess three main functions in response to DNA damage: cell cycle (G1) arrest, stimulation of DNA repair and promotion of cell death (apoptosis). When *p53* is mutated, these mechanisms are lost and the cell can progress as a neoplastic clone. The *p53* acts as a transcription factor, binding to specific sequences of DNA. Mutations can result in clustering of *p53* at its DNA-binding site, causing a loss of function.

The *DCC* gene

The *DCC* (deleted in colon cancer) gene was identified on chromosome 18q21 in 1990 (Madoff, 1998). Both mutations on chromosomes 17 and 18 are found uncommonly in small adenomas but, as the adenomas develop, carcinoma *in situ* changes the incidence rises. The incidence continues to rise with the development of invasive cancer. The loss of heterozygosity on the long arm of chromosome 18 (18q) may be a molecular predictor of a poor prognosis. Loss of one allele occurs in 71 per cent of somatic mutations and in 13 per cent of colorectal cancers. The gene appears to function as a tumour suppressor. This gene has a similarity to a variety of cell-surface glycoproteins including neural cell adhesion molecules. It has been postulated that *DCC*'s effects are a result of abnormal cell matrix or cell–cell interactions. The exact function, however, remains unknown.

The *ras* oncogene

The *ras* family of oncogenes was first identified as the transforming agents in the Harvey and Kirsten murine sarcoma viruses. There are a variety of *ras* oncogenes (H-*ras*, K-*ras*, N-*ras*), which encode for a 21-kDa protein. Activation of *ras* appears, in most cases, to be caused by point mutations usually occurring at codons 12, 13 and 61. These *ras* oncogenes appear to be present in about 50 per cent of colon and rectal tumours. The *ras* mutations by themselves appear, however, to be insufficient to initiate neoplastic change.

The k-*ras* gene is often found mutated in polyps and the incidence appears to rise as the polyp increases in size and dysplastic changes occur. There appears to be no increase, however, as the polyp develops into an invasive malignancy.

The *ras* proteins belong to a large group of nucleotides termed 'guanosine triphosphates'. These proteins appear to play vital roles in the transmission of signals from the cell surface to the nucleus, regulation of the cytoskeleton and cellular proliferation. In normal *ras* expression the proteins alternate between active GTP-bound and inactive GDP-bound states. The mutated *ras* forms remain in the active GTP form. The activated *ras* causes activation of a variety of protein kinases in a cascade-like fashion, which results in the phosphorylation of certain nuclear transcription factors. Some of the activated *ras* functions have also been implicated in the development of angiogenesis factors and the programming of cell death (apoptosis).

Various other genes and oncogenes have been detected, and these are thought to play a role in the development of colorectal cancers (*myc, ras, src*).

Conclusion

The advances that have taken place in the development of molecular biology have provided new insights into the development of colorectal cancers at the molecular level. The historical, epidemiological and histological studies of the adenomatous polyp–cancer sequence are now being revealed at the genetic level. The multistage development of colorectal cancers relies on several classes of genes to be abnormally expressed. These genes include oncogenes, tumour suppressor genes and DNA MMR mechanisms. About 20 per cent of colorectal cancers have a familial link. This implies that some form of inherited element is involved in their development.

The *APC* gene acts as the 'gatekeeper'. The early inactivation of the *APC* gene is detected in the early changes in the development of adenomas but not in the adjacent mucosa. Subsequent gene abnormalities (*p53, DCC, MCC, ras, myc,* DNA repair) accumulate, resulting in a progressive change in the cell clone. K-*ras* mutations also appear to be early events in the neoplastic transformation, with mutations detected in about 50 per cent of adenomas and carcinomas.

The allelic deletions that occur on chromosome 17p usually appear to be late events. The loss of heterozygosity is seen rarely in early oedemas, but in 75 per cent of carcinomas. This finding is similar for changes on 18q (Friend, 1994). Several other chromosomal arms are also found altered, although to lesser degrees. In some 20–50 per cent, changes within regions of chromosomal arms are found in 1q, 4p, 9q and 22q (Fearon et al., 1990).

It would appear that it is the accumulation of gene errors that is critical, and not particularly the specific order in which they occur. The understanding of the various molecular mechanisms in the development of colorectal cancer will, it is hoped, provide new ways of diagnosing and treating the disease based on the molecular mechanisms involved in their aetiology.

References

Aaltonen LA, Peltomaki P, Leach FS, Sistonen P, Pylkkanen L, Mecl JP, Jarvinen H, Powell SM, Jen J, Hamilton SR, et al. (1993) Clues to the pathogenesis of familial colorectal cancer. Science 260: 812-816.

Bishop JM (1981) Oncogenes. Scientific American 140: 69.

Bishop JM (1985) Trends in oncogenes. Trends in Genetics 245-249.

Bishop JM (1987) The molecular genetics of cancer. Science 235: 305-311.

Bodmer W, Bishop T, Karran P (1994) Genetic steps in colorectal cancer. Nature Genetics 6: 217-219.

Bussey HJR (1975) Familial Polyposis Coli. Baltimore: Johns Hopkins University Press.

Cairns J (1981) The origin of human cancers. Nature 289: 353-357.

De Mars R (1969) In: 23rd Annual Symposium Fundamental Cancer Research. Baltimore, Md: Williams & Williams, pp. 105-106.

Duesberg PH (1983) Retroviral transforming genes in normal cells? Nature 304: 219-226.

Fearon ER, Vogelstein BA (1990) A genetic model for colorectal tumorigenesis. Cell 61(Jun): 759-767.

Fearon ER, Cho KR, Nigro JM, Kern SE, Simons JW, Ruppert JM, Hamilton SR, Preisinger AC, Thomas G, Kinzler KW, et al. (1990) Identification of a chromosome 18q gene that is altered in colorectal cancers. Science 247: 49-56.

Friend S (1994) p53: A glimpse at the puppet behind the shadow play. Science 265: 334-335.

Gardner EJ, Richards RC (1953) Multiple cutaneous and subcutaneous lesions occurring simultaneously with hereditary polyposis and osteomatosis. American Journal of Human Genetics 5: 139-147.

Groden J, Thliveris A, Samowitz W, Carlson M, Gelbert L, Albertsen H, Joslyn G, Stevens J, Spirio L, Robertson M, et al. (1991) Identification and characterization of the familial adenomatous polyposis coli gene. Cell 66: 589-600.

Hall NR et al. (1998a) Genetics and the polyp cancer sequence. In: Edelstein PS (ed.), Colon and Rectal Cancer. pp. 3-29.

Hall NR et al. (1998b) Hereditary colorectal cancer syndromes. Seminars in Colon and Rectal Surgery 9: 2-11.

Hamilton SR, Liu B, Parsons RE, Papadopoulos N, Jen J, Powell SM, Krush AJ, Berk T, Cohen Z, Tetu B, et al. (1995) The molecular basis of Turcot's syndrome. New England Journal of Medicine 332: 839-847.

Hamlyn P (1984) Oncogenes. In: Macleod, Sikora (eds), Molecular Biology and Human Disease. pp. 150-163.

Hansen MF, Cavenee WK (1987) Genetics of cancer predisposition. Cancer Research 47: 5518-5527.

Harris CC, Hollstein M (1993) Clinical implications of the p53 tumor-suppressor gene. New England Journal of Medicine 329: 1318-1327.

Ionov Y, Peinado MA, Malkhosyan S, Shibata D, Perucho M (1993) Ubiquitous somatic mutations in simple repeated sequences reveal a new mechanism for colonic carcinogenesis. Nature 363: 558-561.

Kern SE, Pietenpol JA, Thiagalingam S, Seymour A, Kinzler KW, Vogelstein B (1992) Oncogenic forms of p53 inhibit p53-regulated gene expression. Science 256: 827-830.

Kerr JF, Wyllie AH, Currie AR (1972) Apoptosis: basic biological phenomenon with wide-ranging implications in tissue kinetics. British Journal of Cancer 26: 239-257.

Kingsley DM (1994) The TGF-beta superfamily: new members, new receptors and new genetic tests of function in different organisms. Genes and Development 8: 133-146.

Kinzler KW, Nilbert MC, Vogelstein B, Bryan TM, Levy DB, Smith KJ, Preisinger AC, Hamilton SR, Hedge P, Markham A, et al. (1991) Identification of a gene located at chromosome 5q21 that is mutated in colorectal cancers. Science 251: 1366-1370.

Kinzler KW, Vogelstein B (1996) Lessons from hereditary colorectal cancer. Cell 87: 159-170.

Kinzler KW, Vogelstein B (1998) Landscaping the cancer terrain. Science 280: 1036-1037.

Klein G (1981) The role of gene dosage and genetic transpositions in carcinogenesis. Nature 294: 313-318.

Knudson AG Jr (1971) Mutation and cancer: statistical study of retinoblastoma. Proceedings of the National Academy of Sciences of the USA 68: 820-823.

Knudson AG Jr (1985) Hereditary cancer, oncogenes and antioncogenes. Cancer Research 45: 1437-1443.

Lynch HT, Smyrk T, McGinn T, Lanspa S, Cavalieri J, Lynch J, Slominski-Castor S, Cayouette MC, Priluck I, Luce MC (1995) Attenuated familial adenomatous polyposis (AFAP): a phenotypically and genotypically distinctive variant of FAP. Cancer 76: 2427-2433.

Madoff RD (1998) The multistep model of colorectal carcinogenesis. Seminars in Colon and Rectal Surgery 9(1): 30-37.

Markowitz S, Wang J, Myeroff L, Parsons R, Sun L, Lutterbaugh J, Zborowska E, Kinzler KW, Vogelstein B et al. (1995) Inactivation of the type II TGF-beta receptor in colon cancer cells with microsatellite instability. Science 268: 1336-1338.

Marshall C (1984) Viral and cellular genes involved in oncogenesis. Cancer Surveys 3(1): 183-214.

Massague J (1990) The transforming growth factor-beta family. Annual Review of Cell Biology 6: 597-641.

Morin PJ, Vogelstein B, Kinzler KW (1996) Apoptosis and APC in colorectal tumorigenesis. Proceedings of the National Academy of Sciences of the USA 93: 7950-7954.

Nakamura Y (1995) The adenomatous polyposis coli gene and human cancer. Journal of Cancer Research and Clinical Oncology 121: 529-534.

Nordling CO (1953) A new theory on the cancer-inducing mechanism. British Journal of Cancer 7: 68-72.

Northover JM, Murday V (1989) Familial colorectal cancer and familial adenomatous polyposis. Baillière's Clinical Gastroenterology 3: 593-613.

Nowell PC (1960) A minute chromosome in human chronic granulocytic leukaemia. Science 132: 1497.

Nowell PC (1976) The clonal evolution of tumour cell populations: acquired genetic lability permits stepwise selection of variant sublines and underlies tumor progression. Science 194: 23-28.

Parsons R, Myeroff LL, Lui B, Willson JK, Markowitz SD, Kinzler R, Vogelstein B (1995) Microsatellite instability and mutations of the transforming growth factor beta type II receptor gene in colorectal cancer. Cancer Research 55: 5548-5550.

Roberts JAF, Pembrey ME (1985) An Introduction to Medical Genetics. Oxford: Oxford University Press.

Rous P (1911) Transmission of a malignant new growth by means of a cell-free filtrate. Journal of the American Medical Association 198.

Senba S, Konishi F, Okamoto T, Kashiwagi H, Kanazawa K, Miyaki Konishi M, Tsukamoto T (1998) Clinicopathologic and genetic features of non-familial colorectal carcinomas with DNA replication errors. Cancer 82: 279-285.

Souza RF, Appel R, Yin J, Wang S, Smolinski KN, Abraham JM, Zo TT, Shi YQ, Lei J, Cottrell J, Cymes K, Biden K, Simms L, Leggett H, Lynch PM, Frazier M, Powell SM, Harpaz N, Sugimura H, Young J, Meltzer SJ (1996) Microsatellite instability in the insulin-like growth factor II receptor gene in gastrointestinal tumours. Nature Genetics 14: 255-257.

Spirio L, Olschwang S, Groden J, Robertson M, Samowitz W, Joslyn G, Gelbert L, Thliveris A, Carlson M, Otterud B, et al. (1993) Alleles of the APC gene: an attenuated form of familial polyposis. Cell 75: 951–957.

Thibodeau SN, French AJ, Cunningham JM, Tester D, Burgart LJ, Roche PC, McDonnell SK, Schaid DJ, Vockley CW, Michels VV, Far GH, O'Connell MJ (1998) Microsatellite instability in colorectal cancer: different mutator phenotypes and the principal involvement of hMLH1. Cancer Research 58: 1713–1718.

Vogelstein B, Fearon ER, Hamilton SR, Kern SE, Preisinger AC, Leppert M, Nakamura Y, White R, Smits AM, Bos JL (1988) Genetic alterations during colorectal-tumor development. New England Journal of Medicine 319: 525–532.

Weiss RA (1982) RNA Tumour Viruses. Cold Spring Harbor Laboratory, USA .

Glossary

Allele: alternative forms of a gene or DNA sequence that occupy the same site on the chromosome.

Amplification: the production of multiple copies of a sequence of DNA.

Apoptosis: programmed cell death.

Chromosome: genes are linked together to form chromosomes. They are usually in pairs.

Clone: cells arising from a single cell by mitotic division. All these cells have the same genetic constitution.

Desmoid tumour: tumour of connective tissue.

Dominant: the gene produces its effect whether it is present on one or both chromosomes of the pair concerned.

DNA-repair genes: there is continual damage to DNA. These genes act as a 'repair crew'.

Exon: region of a gene transcribed into messenger RNA and translated into protein product.

Gene: segment of DNA that codes for a certain trait.

Genotype: the genetic make-up of an individual.

Locus: site of specific DNA sequence or gene on a chromosome. Different forms of allele (gene) may occupy the locus.

Homozygous: term used when both alleles are identical.

Heterozygous: term used when the two alleles are not identical.

Oncogene: a gene with the potential to cause cancer.

Phenotype: biochemical or physical characteristic reflecting the genetic constitution.

Point mutation: the substitution of a single base-pair in DNA that will affect protein synthesis.

Recessive: the gene produces its effect when it is present on both chromosomes.

Restriction fragments: DNA fragments produced by restriction endonuclease digestion of a sample of DNA.

Restriction fragment length polymorphism: the variation in size of DNA fragments produced by restriction endonuclease digestion caused by variation in DNA sequence at the enzyme recognition site.

Somatic mutation: results in the presence of two different cell lines derived from a single zygote. (Only the descendants of the cell will be affected.)

Translocation: transfer of chromosomal material between two non-homologous chromosomes.

Chapter 3

Colorectal cancer: epidemiology and genetics

Lucy Burgess

Many people have a family member affected by colorectal cancer because it is the second most common cancer in England and Wales (Langman and Boyle, 2002). The causes of the disease are thought mainly to be environmental, such as lifestyle factors. Individuals who are at increased risk include smokers and people who drink alcohol. There is also an increased risk in those who have a diet rich in meat and fat, are overweight and take little exercise. A diet with a high intake of fruit and vegetables has been found to be beneficial in reducing the risk of developing the disease. About 75 per cent of colorectal cancer occurs sporadically (by chance). A family history of colon cancer may increase the likelihood of developing the disease, and about 25 per cent of patients with colorectal cancer may have a genetic contribution and/or similar lifestyle exposure. In about 5 per cent of colon cancer families, germline (found in all cells in the body) gene mutations have been found to be responsible for colon cancer development.

The epidemiological study of colorectal cancer will help to improve knowledge about the aetiology and pathogenesis of the disease and thus potentially improve mortality rates. To reduce the mortality rate from colorectal cancer, treatment outcomes need to be improved and the disease needs to be identified at an earlier and thus more curable stage. Various studies highlight the importance of faecal occult blood testing (FOBT) and sigmoidoscopy in reducing colon cancer mortality. In the USA routine surveillance (colonoscopy at the age of 50) is widely undertaken for individuals at population risk of developing the disease.

The genetic study of the disease contributes to understanding the aetiology, management and treatment of colorectal cancer. Developments in this field will lead to improved identification of those at high risk of the disease and those who may benefit from regular surveillance. In the future, diagnosis of the disease in the absence of symptoms and histological features by the use of genetic markers will allow patients at risk to be identified and treated at an earlier stage. Treatment plans and patient prognosis will be individualized dependent on specific genetic information. Currently a large proportion of the referrals to clinical genetics units in the UK are for families with significant histories of cancer, and those with recognized syndromes such as hereditary non-polyposis colon cancer (HNPCC) and familial adenomatous polyposis (FAP).

Incidence

Colorectal cancer is the fourth most common cancer worldwide and the third most common cancer in the UK after lung and breast cancer, usually occurring in later life. It is the sixth most likely cause of death. Men and women are affected almost equally, with over 783 000 cases annually diagnosed worldwide. Of these, over 401 000 new cases occur in men every year and about 381 000 in women. The incidence in men increases after middle age and this may be attributed to the greater impact of the lifestyle factors on men as they become older. Langman and Boyle (2002) suggest that this may be the result of the more proactive approach of women in seeking earlier investigations that may reveal premalignant lesions such as polyps. Rectal cancer is found to be more common in men (Boyle and Langman, 2001). The lifetime risk of developing a colorectal cancer is thought to be about 5 per cent and 1 in 20 people will develop the disease during his or her lifetime.

In the UK there are 19 000 deaths per year from colorectal cancer (Cancer Outcomes Guidance or COG, 1997). The occurrence of colorectal cancer is about 48 in every 100 000 and incidence increases with age. In England and Wales there are about 25 000 new cases diagnosed each year. Under the age of 45 the incidence is about 2 per 100 000 and over 75 approximately 300 per 100 000.

Colorectal cancer is a disease of older individuals and the average age at which colorectal cancer occurs is 70. The incidence of the disease has increased dramatically since 1975 when the occurrence was approximately 500 000 worldwide. In the UK the incidence has also increased over 25 years; the reasons for this may be because of lifestyle factors and perhaps because more cases of the disease are being detected.

However, although the incidence of colorectal cancer is increasing, deaths from the disease have fallen. This may be because colon cancer is being detected at an earlier stage and/or because treatments have improved.

Worldwide, bowel cancer represents 9.4 per cent of all cancers that occur in men and 10.1 per cent in women. However, the disease is more common in Westernized countries such as the UK, North America and

Europe (excluding eastern Europe), Australia and New Zealand. In these countries, the incidence of colorectal cancer accounts for 12.6 per cent of all cancers and 14.1 per cent in women compared with 7.7 per cent in men and 7.9 per cent in women in other areas.

Atkin (2002) argues that a population surveillance programme should exist because the disease fulfils most of the World Health Organization (WHO) screening criteria. Also many lives could be saved, because if patients are treated at premalignant adenoma stage the disease is almost 100 per cent curable. Currently 60 per cent of the cases diagnosed are cured.

Survival

Every year 394 000 deaths occur from colorectal cancer, and bowel cancer is the second most common cause of cancer deaths in European men. Differences in survival rates are apparent in the UK, Europe and the USA. This may be related to treatment modalities or the stage of disease at presentation. Five-year survival rates in the UK are worse than in Europe. In the UK, individuals with bowel cancer survive for about three years after diagnosis, dependent on the stage of the disease. Overall, women also tend to survive for longer than men.

Deprivation has been linked to survival from colorectal cancer. Individuals from more deprived backgrounds have lower rates of survival than those from more prosperous circumstances. Deprivation may include social deprivation as well as material aspects. Furthermore, deprivation rather than just poverty is linked to aspects of survival; the reasons for this require further research.

Survival rates vary with the stage of the disease; this is outlined in Table 3.1.

Table 3.1 Stage and survival from colorectal cancer (Hardy et al., 2001)

TNM classification	Stage	Survival rate (%)
Stage 0	Pre-Dukes' A	100
Stage 1 (T_1 or T_2, N_0, M_0)	Dukes' A	80
Stage 2 (T_3 or T_4), N_0, M_0	Dukes' B	45
Stage 3 (any T, N_1, M_0)	Dukes' C	30
Stage 4 (distant metastases)	Dukes' D	< 5

Environmental influences on the development of colorectal cancer

Environmental factors are known to influence the development of the disease in about 70–80 per cent of all individuals who develop cancer. Essentially, most these cancers may be preventable. Environmental factors such as lifestyle, social and cultural factors are difficult to quantify but may help explain why the incidence in the UK is greater than in other culturally different countries. The influence of the environment can be seen in individuals from non-Westernized countries who settle in Westernized communities. If they adopt the lifestyle of the community they go on to develop colorectal cancer at rates similar to that of the indigenous population. The suggestion that environmental factors play a large part in the aetiology of colorectal cancer has been highlighted by Boyle et al. (2001). They describe that the risk for developing colorectal cancer in adult children of Japanese individuals who have emigrated to the USA is the same as that of the general population in the USA. Indeed this is three to four times higher than in Japanese individuals living in Japan.

Causal factors

Animal fat and meat intake

The development of colorectal cancer may be influenced by dietary fat and meat intake, which constitutes a major part of the Western diet, although the evidence is not without question. Willet's epidemiological study (Willetts et al., 1990) of 88 751 female nurses aged 34–59 in the USA highlights this issue. Entry criteria for the study participants specified that they should be free of inflammatory bowel disease or cancer. The women were studied over 10 years and their intake of animal fats and other lifestyle issues were analysed. The consumption of animal fats was found to be associated with an increased risk of colon cancer. This research confirms recommendations that meats high in fat should be substituted by fish or chicken, which contain less fat.

Overall dietary fat intake has been shown to increase the risk of developing benign polyps or colorectal cancer moderately (Chyou et al., 1996). However, Boyle and Langman (2002) suggest that such studies may be unsubstantiated and that dietary fat may not be of such importance in the development of colorectal cancer as previously expected. They do, however, comment that dietary fat intake could affect the secretion of bile salts and that this might affect the epithelial lining of the colon.

Protein

Protein intake has been found to affect the levels of procarcinogens in the body. Alternatively, carcinogens produced when meat is burnt during cooking could be ingested (Langman and Boyle, 2002). Secondary bile acids (Langman and Boyle, 2002) and the cooking of meat have potentially been identified as carcinogens. Studies are inconclusive; however, clearer links have been found between animal-based protein and intestinal cancer or polyp development. Giovannucci et al. (1994) confirms that the correlation between colorectal cancer and protein intake is more marked than for fat intake.

Fruit, vegetables and fibre

Studies have identified the protective properties of fruit, vegetables and fibre. There have been discussions about which type of fibre is the most beneficial. Fruit and vegetable fibre contains soluble, degradable constituents such as pectin and plant gum, whereas cereal fibre consists of insoluble, non-degradable components. The intake of fibre has been linked to faecal bulk and transit time. If faeces are kept in the colon for a longer than average length of time, there is a chance that toxins may build up, e.g. colonic bacteria produce toxic waste and colon cancer may be linked to prolonged exposure to these toxins. Communities that consume higher levels of fibre have lower rates of colorectal cancer. This has been highlighted as a contributory factor in the difference in incidence of colorectal cancer occurring between Africa and Westernized countries. In particular, the intake of vegetable and fruit fibre, rather than cereal fibre, is thought to be protective. This may be because there are factors other than fibre in fruit and vegetables that increase this effect.

Fruit and vegetables are a rich source of the antioxidant vitamin C. Antioxidants inactivate free radicals, harmful molecules that are produced by the body and have been associated with the development of cancer (Saffrey and Stewart, 1997). Furthermore, fruit and vegetables also provide folate, which is important for DNA function (this could be an important factor in the expression, i.e. the 'switching on', of genes). Indeed protection from colon cancer and polyps in individuals with higher intakes of fruit and vegetables has been demonstrated by Bird et al. (1995), probably as a result of the increase in folate levels.

Physical activity, body mass index and energy intake

Physical activity is thought to decrease the risk of colorectal cancer. Studies have highlighted that men who are physically active have lower levels of disease occurrence (Giovannucci et al., 1994). This association is apparent even after other factors such as body mass index (BMI) and diet have been taken into account. Regular physical activity such as brisk walking has been shown to decrease the occurrence of large adenomas in the distal colon. This is thought to be because of the decreased intestinal transit time which allows potential carcinogens to have shorter contact with the mucosa of the gut. Prostaglandins and antioxidant enzymes are affected by physical activity but it is not known if these substances have an influential role in the development of colorectal cancer.

Obesity

The evidence to support the link between obesity and colorectal cancer is unclear (Boyle et al., 2001). However, a link has been shown between obesity and adenoma development. The ability of individuals to use energy efficiently may influence the increased risk of cancer associated with overeating. Thus, the risk of colorectal cancer development may be lower in those individuals with a more efficient metabolism.

Smoking

The effect of smoking on the development of colorectal cancer is unclear and indeed the effect of the interaction between smoking and alcohol on the development of cancer is hard to separate. Giovannucci et al. (1994) and Baron et al. (1994) report that the incidence of colorectal cancer is increased among those who smoke. The reasons for this need further investigation; however, Boyle and Langman (2002) suggest that the increased risk of benign polyps found in smokers may contribute to this picture. Furthermore, the Nurses Health Study, among others, has highlighted the contributions of diet, smoking, low folate intake and alcohol to the development of benign hyperplastic colonic polyps, premalignant lesions such as adenomatous polyps, and colorectal cancer.

Alcohol

Alcohol is responsible for the increased risk of developing the disease, even when the effects of smoking for individuals with both risk factors are removed. Boyle and Langman (2002) suggest that the evidence is unclear about whether the effect of alcohol intake is direct or whether it is the effect of alcohol on folate removal (useful in cancer prevention) that is the significant factor.

Occupation/industrial exposure

There have been no conclusive studies to date.

Lifestyle issues

Boyle and Langman (2001) suggest that lifestyle factors, such as dietary intake, smoking and alcohol, are often seen to be the responsibility of the individual and thus blame may be attributed if the disease develops. They argue that these choices may not be solely the responsibility of the individual and that Government legislation could do much more to encourage lifestyles that decrease cancer risk. Indeed, currently the Government, as part of the plan to reduce cancer, is offering fruit to schoolchildren as part of this message.

Chemoprevention

The role of non-steroidal anti-inflammatory drugs and aspirin

Individuals who take non-steroidal anti-inflammatory drugs (NSAIDs) are at a reduced risk of developing colorectal cancer (Peleg et al., 1994). This may be because they protect against colon cancer development by inducing cell death or by inhibiting growth in colon cancer cell lines; this may be the result of the action of protecting against the effects of cyclo-oxygenase 2 (COX-2) upregulation, which is seen in colonic tumours. Hirota et al. (1996) confirm the effect of NSAIDs on polyp development in patients with familial adenomatous polyposis coli, in that fewer and smaller polyps develop in individuals treated with NSAIDs.

Trials are ongoing into the use of aspirin and insoluble starch in chemoprevention, including the Concerted Action in Polyposis Prevention trials CAPP 1 and CAPP 2. Langman and Boyle (2000) comments that risk reduction attributable to taking aspirin may be in the region of 30–40 per cent for adenoma and carcinoma development. Aspirin may also play a part in the reduction of the incidence of stomach and oesophageal cancer.

Hormone replacement therapy

Newcomb and Storer (1995) highlight the reduction in risk of the development of colorectal cancer in women who take hormone replacement therapy (HRT) over 5–10 years. Taking HRT over periods longer than 10 years appears to reduce the effect of the drug on the development of colorectal cancer and therefore is less beneficial than when taken for between five and 10 years. However, this effect has not been seen in women under the age of 50. The evidence is contentious and may be explained by the effect of HRT on DNA methylation (switching genes on or off). Oestrogen receptors have been found in the lining of the bowel – a fact that may explain some of the findings. However, tamoxifen (the anti-oestrogen) has not been shown to influence the development of large bowel cancers and the contraceptive pill does not appear to have the same protective effect as HRT.

Further studies are needed to ascertain the significance of HRT on the development of colorectal cancer before it is offered to women at increased risk of colorectal cancer to lower their chance of developing the disease. Also, as HRT may influence the development of breast cancer this needs to be weighed against the potential decrease in colorectal cancer development.

Calcium and vitamin D

Reduced levels of colon cancer are found in individuals who are exposed to sunlight (Emerson and Weiss, 1992). Garland et al. (1989) comment that lower levels of serum vitamin D have been found to be related to lower levels of colon cancer risk. It has been suggested that vitamin D receptors are found in the colon and that the vitamin has been shown to reduce the rate of colon cancer cell multiplication. Boyle and Langman (2001) suggest that a high calcium diet may be protective because calcium may counteract the carcinogenic properties of high fat meat by binding free bile and fatty acids.

Antioxidants

Vitamins A, C and E

It has been suggested that these vitamins may protect against the formation of adenomas. However, vitamin A has been suggested as increasing the risk of individuals developing lung cancer, and this picture is also apparent in colon cancer because vitamin D, via retinoids, interferes with the suppression of cell multiplication.

Reduction in the risk of colorectal cancer (Boyle and Langman, 2001)

- Eat plenty of fruit and vegetables (five portions a day)
- Diet low in animal fat
- Reduce red meat intake and replace with fish or poultry

- Moderate alcohol intake
- Avoid smoking
- Regular exercise – such as brisk walking
- Maintain a healthy weight
- Participate in population screening programmes as available
- Seek advice about symptoms including prolonged change in bowel habits without explanation, rectal bleeding, abdominal pain and a feeling of fullness after defecation, etc.

Individuals at increased risk

All cancers are genetic in origin, in that damage to genes is responsible for the development of the cancer. Only about 5 per cent of patients have cancers that are linked to a genetic syndrome in which there is a germline mutation (i.e. there is a gene fault in every cell in the body). Examples of this include FAP and HNPCC, and the genes causing these conditions have been identified. A germline mutation can be inherited in families and can be passed from father to son and mother to daughter. About 25 per cent of cancers occur in family clusters and may be caused by other genes that have not yet been discovered, several interacting genes (polygenic), multifactorial mechanisms and environmental/lifestyle factors or chance. About 70 per cent of patients have no positive or negative factors known to predispose to the development of colorectal cancer and thus are sporadic cases probably occurring by chance and lifestyle issues (Figure 3.1).

Figure 3.1 Cancer arises from gene faults and all cancer is genetic in origin.

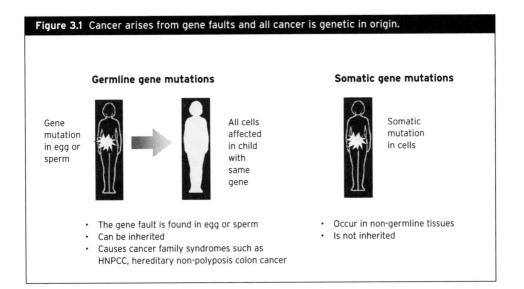

Germline gene mutations

Gene mutation in egg or sperm

All cells affected in child with same gene

Somatic gene mutations

Somatic mutation in cells

- The gene fault is found in egg or sperm
- Can be inherited
- Causes cancer family syndromes such as HNPCC, hereditary non-polyposis colon cancer

- Occur in non-germline tissues
- Is not inherited

When assessing the significance of a family history it is important to determine:

- the number of relatives affected
- whether they are first-/second-degree relatives, etc.
- age at which the colorectal cancer occurred
- whether anyone in the family had more than one primary cancer
- whether there are any other cancers in the family that could be linked to an inherited colon cancer syndrome such as endometrial cancer, etc. (see 'HNPCC' below).

The risk of colorectal cancer is shown in Table 3.2.

Table 3.2 Risk of colorectal cancer (CRC)

	Lifetime risk (%)
General population	5
Personal family history of CRC (tubulovillous ademonas, etc.)	15-20
Inflammatory bowel disease	15-40
Hereditary non-polyposis colon cancer mutation (HNPCC)	70-80
Familial adenomatous polyposis (FAP)	95

Family history, FAP and HNPCC

Family history

Individuals with a positive family history that does not match the HNPCC criteria and those who have a first-degree relative with the cancer have an increased lifetime risk of developing cancer (see Table 3.3).

Table 3.3 Recognition of significant family histories

Two, three or more of the same cancers (e.g. colorectal) in families

Early age of onset of tumours

Individuals with two or more primary tumours, such as two colorectal primaries, or a colorectal and separate endometrial primary cancer

Family members with histories of colorectal adenocarcinomas, endometrial, stomach or ovarian tumours

Cole and Sleightholme (2002)

When there are two or more affected individuals within a family, the likelihood that this could be an inherited cancer is increased. The younger the individuals affected, or the greater number of affected individuals, the greater the relative risk (this is the risk of a particular individual developing cancer compared with the general population). Explanations for this may include genes with lower penetrance (this is the incidence of cancer occurring in an individual with a known fault) than in adenomatous polyposis coli (APC)/mismatch repair (MMR) genes, environmental/lifestyle factors, coincidence and multifactoral interactions between environment and genetic factors. Evidence to support screening programmes is based on the fact that, in the case of colorectal surveillance, screening the average risk population reduces the risk of dying from colorectal cancer, although evidence to ascertain the benefit of other surveillance is limited (Cole et al., 2002); however, some guidelines are discussed in Table 3.4. The lifetime risk of colorectal cancer in a first-degree relative of a patient with the disease is shown in Table 3.5.

Table 3.4 Current family history screening guidelines

Inclusion criteria (Cole and Sleightholme, 2002)	Screening method	Age range for screening (years)	Dunlop guidelines (2002)
One first-degree relative[a] Aged > 40	Reassure, give general advice regarding healthy lifestyle and symptoms	Not applicable	One first-degree relative aged > 45 - reassure
Aged < 40	Colonoscopy every 5 years, appointment at local screening unit	25-65, or 5 years before cancer if later	One first degree relative aged < 45 Initial colonoscopy at age 35 and repeat at age 55
Two first-degree relatives[b] Average age > 70	Reassure, give general advice about healthy lifestyle and symptoms	Not applicable	
Average age 60-70	Single colonoscopy, appointment at local screening unit	About 55	Initial colonoscopy at age 35 and if clear repeat at age 55
Average age 50-60	Colonoscopy every 5 years, appointment at local screening unit	30-65	Initial colonoscopy at age 35 and if clear repeat at age 55
Average age < 50	Colonoscopy every 3-5 years, referral to genetics unit	30-65	Initial colonoscopy at age 35 and if clear repeat at age 55

Table 3.4 Current family history screening guidelines (contd)

Inclusion criteria (Cole and Sleightholme, 2002)	Screening method	Age range for screening (years)	Dunlop guidelines (2002)
Three close relatives but not meeting Amsterdam criteria	Colonoscopy every 3-5 years: referral to clinical genetics unit	30-40: stop at 65	
Three close relatives meeting Amsterdam criteria	Colonoscopy every 2 years: referral to clinical genetics unit Depending on family history other screening may be required	25-65	2-yearly colonoscopy and gastroscopy (aged 50 or 5 years before earliest gastric cancer)
HNPCC gene carrier	Colonoscopy every 2 years: Gynaecological surveillance (if applicable) Urinary tract surveillance ? Upper gastrointestinal surveillance	25-65	
Familial adenomatous polyposis	Annual sigmoidoscopy Referral to genetics unit	Age 12 onwards	Annual sigmoidoscopy and oesophago-gastroduodenoscopy

a   A first-degree relative is a brother/sister, father/mother or child.
b   Two first-degree relatives are first degree to each other such as a mother and grandmother, mother and her brother and one must be first degree to the patient.

Average age: if two or more relatives are affected, average the age to determine the screening category, e.g. one relative affected aged 60 and one aged 70 = average age of 65.

Table 3.5 Lifetime risk of colorectal cancer in a first-degree relative of a patient with colorectal cancer (CRC)

	Lifetime risk of developing CRC
General population (no family history)	1 in 35 (3%)
One first-degree relative aged > 45 affected	1 in 17 (6%)
One first-degree and one second-degree relative affected	1 in 12 (8%)
One first-degree aged < 45 affected	1 in 10 (10%)
Two first-degree relatives affected	1 in 6 (17%)
More than two first-degree relatives affected	1 in 3
Autosomal dominant pedigree (such as in HNPCC, etc.)	1 in 2
HNPCC gene mutation carrier	70-80%
FAP gene mutation carrier	100%

Houlston et al. (1990) after Lovett (1976)   HPNCC, hereditary non-polyposis colon cancer

In families in which colorectal cancer is not associated with HNPCC or FAP syndromes, the genetic events leading to cancer development are as described in Chapter 2.

High risk

Familial adenomatous polyposis (Figure 3.2)

This condition accounts for about 1 per cent of all colorectal cancers and is an autosomal dominant genetic condition in which almost all individuals who carry the gene develop over 100 adenomatous polyps which, if untreated, develop into colorectal cancer (Burlow, 1987).

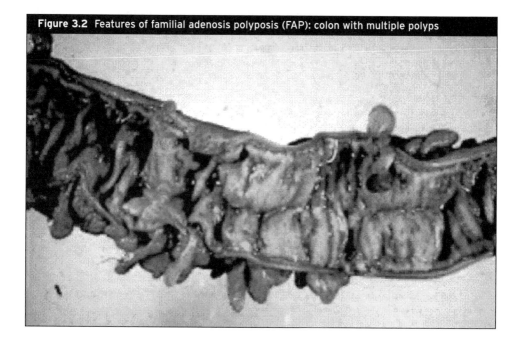

Figure 3.2 Features of familial adenosis polyposis (FAP): colon with multiple polyps

The average time for development of colon cancer is about 30 years, and by the age of 14 most gene carriers will have some polyps. In most gene carriers (70–80 per cent), the causative gene, *APC*, can be identified. Other tumours and features can occur within FAP and include upper gastrointestinal polyps, brain tumours, hepatoblastoma, desmoid tumours (locally invasive fibromatous tumours), adrenal adenomas, and benign craniofacial and long-bone tumours, papillary thyroid cancer, periampullary carcinoma and CHRPE (congenital hypertrophy of the retinal pigment epithelium).

A variation of FAP, attenuated FAP, accounts for fewer polyps, later onset of cancer and lower penetrance (not all individuals with the gene fault will develop cancer).

IF FAP is identified, an extensive family history should be taken, although in 30 per cent of cases new mutations will be identified and thus no other family members will be obviously affected. Cole et al. (2002) recommend that the parents of newly identified affected individuals should undergo a single colonoscopy to ascertain whether they may be affected by attenuated FAP. Surveillance recommendations for potentially affected individuals include annual flexible sigmoidoscopy (because the polyps occur obviously in the left side of the colon) and/or colonoscopy from the age of 12 to the age of 40, or until the individual undergoes genetic testing to detect whether they carry the mutated gene.

Several studies have shown that morbidity and mortality in FAP can be reduced by identifying gene carriers, bowel surveillance and surgery (Vasen et al., 1990). If the surveillance reveals that the individual has polyps, prophylactic surgery may be recommended. This includes ileorectal anastomosis and reconstruction of the rectal pouch using the small bowel. Evidence is available to illustrate that mutations in the second half of the gene may result in earlier cancer development and therefore, in this group, restorative colectomy is recommended.

After surgery there is still a risk of other tumours, especially peri-ampullary and papillary tumours, and there are issues about the potential benefit of upper gastrointestinal surveillance to observe for upper duodenal polyps. However, the benefit of surveillance is difficult to assess because indeed the mortality and morbidity rates associated with major pancreaticoduodenal resection, when duodenal polyps have been detected, are high (Dunlop, 2002). In families where there is a known gene mutation, there is controversy over the timing of identification of the gene fault in children (molecular analysis), although it is usually undertaken at around the age that surveillance should begin. On the positive side, if individuals are not gene mutation carriers they will be spared the need to undergo annual sigmoidoscopy and if they are gene mutation carriers surgical intervention can be planned to reduce colorectal cancer risk as soon as is practical.

In a family where an *APC* gene fault has been identified and an individual does not carry the gene fault, that person is then at population risk of developing a colorectal cancer and thus on-going bowel surveillance is not required.

An alteration in the *APC* gene (11307K) has been identified in about 6 per cent of the Ashkenazai Jewish population that doubles colorectal cancer risk. It is important to ascertain cultural background to determine whether genetic testing for this mutation is appropriate because this can be undertaken in a family member without the need to analyse the DNA of an affected individual.

CAPP 1

A trial (Concerted Action in Polyposis Prevention – CAPP 1) (Burn et al., 1995) is currently determining the role of chemoprophylaxis in the role of development of polyps using aspirin and resistant or digestible starch. Entry criteria include being a gene carrier of the *APC* gene fault or having FAP and the features of the disease and an intact colon.

The patient is allocated to one of four groups to take the following on a daily basis:

1. Aspirin and resistant starch
2. Placebo and resistant starch
3. Aspirin and digestible starch
4. Placebo and digestible starch.

Assessment is undertaken by endoscopy and recorded on a yearly basis to examine the number, size, location and histology of polyps present in the bowel.

APC mutation-positive family
An example of such a family is shown in Figure 3.3.

Other autosomal dominant conditions predisposing to colon and other cancers

Peutz–Jegher syndrome
Patients with this syndrome have an increased risk of cancers of the breast, endometrium, pancreas, ovaries and testes as well as of the intestine. This is a rare syndrome and the patient may have features that include black or blue melanin spots on the skin and gastrointestinal polyps. Patients with this syndrome should be referred to their local clinical genetics unit for advice and screening recommendations.

Turcot's syndrome
In this rare syndrome, besides multiple colonic polyps, patients may have brain tumours. The syndrome is the result of faults in the *APC* and *HNPCC* genes. Patients and relatives should be referred to the clinical genetics unit for assessment, and regular colonoscopic surveillance will be recommended.

Juvenile polyposis
In this condition numerous polyps occur in the colon, stomach and small intestine. There may also be other features, including learning difficulties, heart disease, etc. Surveillance is recommended and colectomy may be advised.

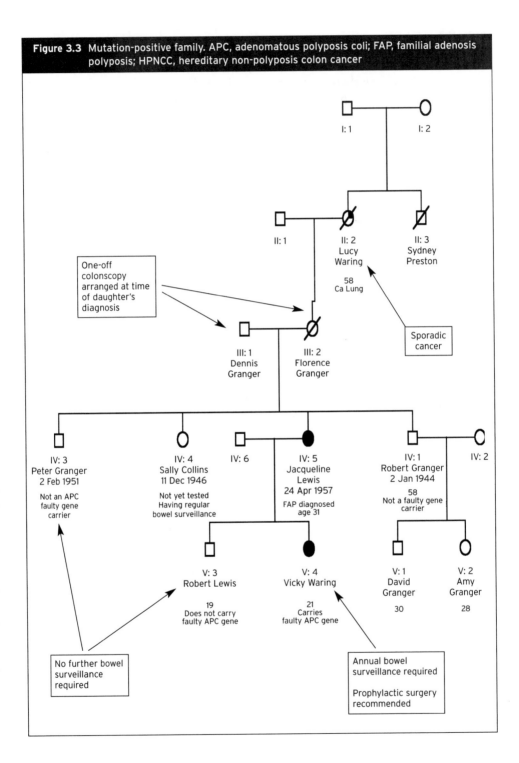

Figure 3.3 Mutation-positive family. APC, adenomatous polyposis coli; FAP, familial adenosis polyposis; HPNCC, hereditary non-polyposis colon cancer

Recessively inherited colorectal cancer (MYH/MAP)

An inherited bowel cancer syndrome called MYH associated polyposis or MAP has recently been discovered. For cancer to occur, the individual needs a faulty copy of the gene from both parents. Features of the condition include 20–30 or more bowel polyps.

Hereditary non-polyposis colorectal cancer

It is important to identify individuals who may fall into high-risk families, such as with HNPCC (Lynch et al., 1993), where a gene fault may be identifiable. HNPCC is a condition in which polyps can occur in the bowel (despite the term 'non-polyposis') and there may be a fairly rapid progression to colorectal cancer. In addition to colon cancer, other cancers may also occur including renal tract transitional cell carcinoma, ovarian cancer, small bowel adenoma and endometrial cancer. Approximate rates of incidence are described in Table 3.6.

Table 3.6 Rates of incidence of tumours in HNPCC

Tumour	Approximate incidence in HNPCC (%)
Colorectal cancer:	
Male aged 50-70	45-70
Female aged 50-70	20-35
Endometrial: age 50-70	10-40
Small bowel adenocarcinoma	1-2
Stomach	1-12
Ovarian	1-6

HPNCC, hereditary non-polyposis colon cancer

Various criteria for identifying HNPCC have been recommended (Table 3.7). Syngal et al. (2000) suggest that, if the modified Amsterdam criteria shown in Table 3.8 are used, HNPCC represents 3–5 per cent of colorectal cancers.

Table 3.7 Amsterdam criteria

Three or more cases of colorectal cancer
A minimum of two generations affected
One first-degree relative of the other two affected
One case diagnosed before the age of 50
FAP excluded

FAP, familial adenosis polyposis

Table 3.8 Modified Amsterdam criteria

Modified Amsterdam	Amsterdam II	Bethesda
In adjusting for smaller families – can include just two cases of colorectal cancer (one diagnosed younger than 55)	Can substitute other HNPCC-related cancers, e.g. small bowel, renal tract transitional cell carcinoma	Amsterdam criteria
Two colorectal cancers and either endometrial cancer or other early onset cancer		Any two HNPCC-related cancers
		Patients with colorectal cancers, one < 45 years or adenoma < 40 years
		Patient with colorectal cancer or endometrial cancer < 45 years
		Specific colorectal cancer histology
		Adenoma < 40 years

HPNCC, hereditary non-polyposis colon cancer

Mutations in genes causing these cancers have been identified as *MLH1*, *MSH2*, *MSH6*, *PMS1* and *PMS2* and are MMR (mismatch repair) genes. Genetic testing is currently routinely available for *MLH1* and *MSH2* and *MSH6*. Testing for other genes involved may be available on a research basis. A typical HNPCC family tree is shown in Figure 3.4.

Mismatch repair genes (*MLH1*, *MSH2*)

These genes recognize and repair DNA mismatches, by binding mismatches, separating, destroying and re-synthesizing new DNA strands. When there is a germline fault in an MMR gene the individual is more susceptible to cancer (Figure 3.5).

Guidelines for screening in HNPCC families are often based on colorectal screening and on the types of tumours found within a particular family. Recommendations for surveillance other than colonoscopy vary widely and will depend on individual family histories (Burt, 2000).

Colon screening

Guidelines for bowel screening recommend the use of colonoscopy because of the incidence of right-sided tumours. Frequency of screening

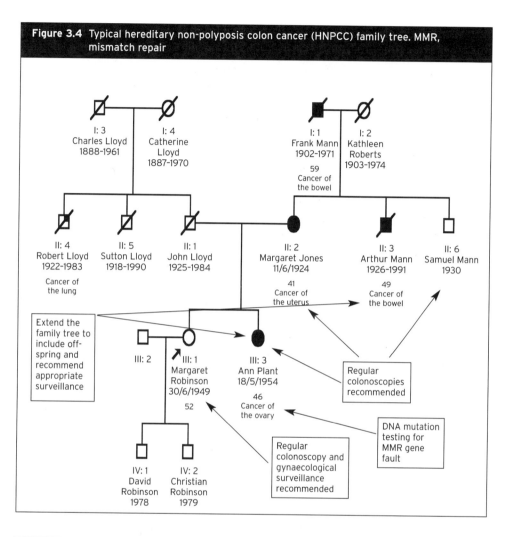

Figure 3.4 Typical hereditary non-polyposis colon cancer (HNPCC) family tree. MMR, mismatch repair

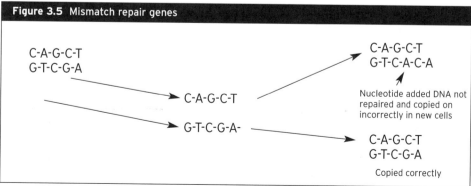

Figure 3.5 Mismatch repair genes

recommended is 1- to 3-yearly commencing at age 25–30 years, although this will vary depending on family history, risk to the individual, patient age, available resources and local guidelines (Burt, 2000). The disadvantages of screening include cost, complications and potential non-compliance. Prophylactic colectomy may be considered by some asymptomatic gene mutation carriers (Vasen et al., 1996). Vasen et al. (1998) provide evidence of the benefit of surveillance in gene carriers versus treatment for colorectal cancer in gene carriers in terms of cost–benefit, morbidity and mortality in families.

Gynaecological screening
Women who are gene carriers of MMR genes are at a 40 per cent lifetime risk of developing endometrial cancer and may be at greater risk of developing endometrial cancer than colon cancer. Annual transvaginal ultrasonography and/or annual hysteroscopy/endometrial biopsy may be recommended. Cole et al. (2002) argue that there is little evidence to support this programme and, as the survival rate from endometrial cancer is high, routine surveillance may not alter the detection of this cancer. Transvaginal ultrasonography (and CA125 measurements) will, however, also be of benefit in the assessment of the ovaries, because ovarian cancer incidence is also increased in HNPCC carriers; however, evidence to support this surveillance procedure is also lacking. Some female gene carriers may opt for hysterectomy and bilateral Salpingo oophrectomy that substantially reduces their risk of developing endometrial or ovarian cancer. Surveillance for women in families where mutations are not known is difficult to assess, particularly where gynaecological tumours are obvious in the family tree.

Other surveillance
Dependent on the family history, other cancer surveillance may be recommended, such as urological or gastric surveillance.

CAPP 2

CAPP 2 is an ongoing trial to ascertain the effect of aspirin and starch on the development of polyps in patients who have HNPCC and/or are mutation carriers. Patients undergoing treatment for cancer are excluded initially. The patients take combinations of aspirin and starch and placebos for two years, and are assessed endoscopically for adenoma development, size, location and histology on a 1- to 2-yearly basis. The objective of the trial is to determine whether taking aspirin and/or resistant starch reduces adenoma development and progression in a genetically predisposed population.

Genetic instability

Genetic instability can occur in colorectal cancer and other cancers.

Microsatellite instability (MSI) in tumour tissue occurs as a result of DNA MMR faults that lead to errors in nucleotide (microsatellite) repeats in the genes.

In individuals where there is tumour MSI (also called RER – replication error), the chance that there is a mutation in a DNA MMR gene in the germline (present in every cell in the body not just in tumour tissue) is greatly increased.

In practice, tumour tissue may be examined from patients under the age of 35 who have colorectal cancer years or who have a moderate or strong family history of colorectal and/or muscinous ovarian and/or endometrial cancers to observe for MSI. If this is identified, germline DNA (from a blood sample) can be examined for *MLH1*, *MSH2* or *MSH6* gene faults because there is a greatly increased likelihood that these will be found, which can lead to cancers occurring in HNPCC (Farrington et al., 1998). Immunohistochemistry studies may also be undertaken in conjunction with MSI studies. Lack of staining indicates that MMR gene expression may be absent and is a useful tool in identifying whether to test for germline *MLH1*, *MSH2* or *MSH6* mutation.

This unstable genomic factor may be contributory to the development of cancer, and indeed factors such as the type and extent of the changes may greatly contribute to future understanding, diagnosis and treatment of the disease.

Epigenetic events

These are changes occurring during cell division that do not happen as a result of changes in the DNA sequence. This includes whether or not genes are activated (expressed). Other ongoing research includes studies of 'imprinting', a mechanism by which the paternal copy of a gene may be expressed differently to the maternal copy of a gene. If there is a loss of imprinting, there may be an increased activation of growth factors or the silencing of tumour suppressor genes, which may lead to the development of cancer. These types of changes may make the colonic mucosa more susceptible to the development of cancer and could be used to identify high-risk individuals when biopsies of colon cells appear normal.

Autosomal dominant inheritance and the two-hit theory

Gene mutations known to lead to HNPCC and FAP are usually inherited autosomal dominantly. This means that it takes only one faulty copy of the gene for the disease to develop. However, the mechanism for the development of cancer is slightly different in that usually, if there is a remaining normal copy of a gene pair, this will be working to provide protection against cancer development. It is only after a second hit (Knudson's hypothesis) as a result of an environmental event that cancer may perhaps develop. A faulty gene may be inherited from either mother or father.

Penetrance

In individuals who carry a faulty MMR gene, not all will develop cancer because of the issue of penetrance. Thus in some families cancer will appear to skip a generation. The issue of penetrance means that an individual can be a faulty gene carrier without developing the disease, because of other mechanisms that are at work within the body. These include modifying genes, the influence of the environment and other factors. However, most individuals with a faulty gene will develop cancer at some point during their lives.

Figure 3.6 (a) How is it inherited? (b) What if the gene is inherited?

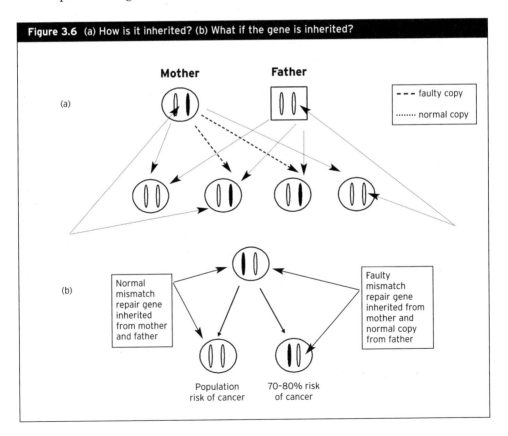

Family history and other factors increasing risk

Table 3.9 summarizes these issues.

Table 3.9 Factors increasing risk

Element increasing risk	Percentage of all CRC cases
Family history	15-20
Hereditary non-polyposis colon cancer	5
Familial polyposis coli	1
Irritable bowel disease	1
Coeliac disease	> 1

Previous colorectal cancer

Individuals at increased risk of colorectal cancer development include those who have previously had a colorectal cancer. In addition, radiotherapy to the pelvic region for treatment of gynaecological cancer or benign disease increases the risk of rectosigmoidal cancer development, usually about 10 years after the completion of treatment.

Inflammatory bowel syndrome

Inflammatory bowel disease is also believed to increase the risk.

Ulcerative colitis

Severe ulcerative colitis over a period of 2–8 years is associated with an increased risk of colorectal cancer. Hardy (2002) suggests that cancers may arise in individuals with dysplastic changes; however, the significance of the grade of dysplastic changes and subsequent development of cancer is difficult to assess. Furthermore, studies have shown that before recognizable dysplastic changes in the mucosa are apparent, molecular changes have already occurred, e.g. MSI, *TP53* mutations and chromosomal instability investigations in non-dysplastic mucosa have been identified.

Sporadic adenomatous polyps

Individuals who develop adenomatous polyps are at increased risk of developing a colorectal cancer.

Family clusters of cancer

About 25 per cent of all cases of colorectal cancer occur in family clusters, which may be caused by common lifestyle factors and/or genes that have yet to be identified, or chance. The family histories do not fit the pattern of HNPCC and FAP. However, additional screening is recommended because the risk to individuals, dependent on number of relatives, age of relatives, etc., is increased.

Family history clinics

Patients with family histories of cancer are often seen in family history clinics and may be referred to symptomatic services or to local clinical genetic units.

Guidelines for referral will vary, but are usually similar to those in Table 3.10. In the West Midlands the West Midlands Family Cancer Strategy (WMFACS) (Cole and Sleightholme, 2000) has been in use, by this model; using a family history questionnaire low-risk patients are triaged out at primary care level and patients with a moderate- or high-risk family history are forwarded to the service. After consent to search records and notes, histological confirmation is obtained if possible and consultant review is undertaken. Histological confirmation is important because 'stomach cancers' reported in family histories may be confirmed as colon, endometrial or ovarian. This information is important because it may alter assessment of family history and management recommendations. Those in moderate-risk categories are entered on to the database and the recommendations are fed back to the relevant professional, often a nurse specialist in their local hospital. More information about this can be found on the following website (www.bwhct.nhs.uk).

The nurse specialist will be able to follow the consultant advice given, and if other family information comes to light make his or her own assessment of

Table 3.10 Guidelines for referral

One first-degree relative aged under 45 affected[a]
One first-degree and one-second degree relative with average age of under 70 affected[b]
Two first-degree relatives with an average age of under 70 affected[a]
More than two first-degree relatives affected
HNPCC gene mutation carrier
FAP gene mutation carrier

[a]A first-degree relative is mother, father, brother or sister. Two first-degree relatives for clarity can be defined as one first-degree relative to the patient and one first-degree relative to the affected relative, e.g. father and grandfather to the patient.
[b]Average age, e.g. one relative of 72 and one relative of 66 = an average age of 69.
FAP, familial adenosis polyposis; HPNCC, hereditary non-polyposis colon cancer.

the patient's risk. At the moderate-risk consultation the nurse specialist will:

- explore patient's past medical history, check for symptoms (such as change of bowel habits, rectal bleeding, if symptomatic – urgent investigations may be required), information regarding lifestyle, anxieties and worries, etc.
- extend the pedigree to add other individuals such as siblings and children of affected individuals, who may also require surveillance at a current or a later date
- clarify types of cancer, polyps and ages of cancer occurrence
- discuss screening type and frequency
- consider storing or asking for consent of relatives to store DNA (from a blood sample) or for consent for tumour tissue studies from previously removed cancer tissue
- discuss relevant lifestyle and health recommendations based on relevant research.

An example is illustrated in Figure 3.7.

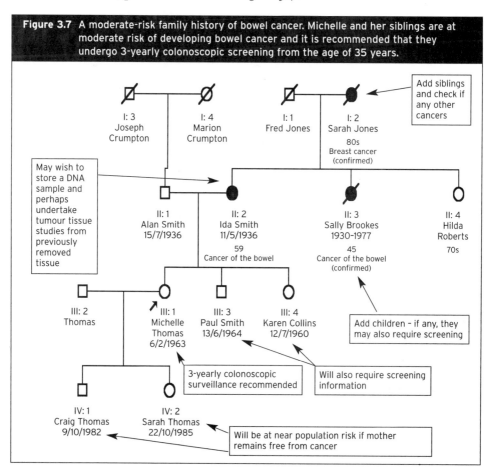

Figure 3.7 A moderate-risk family history of bowel cancer. Michelle and her siblings are at moderate risk of developing bowel cancer and it is recommended that they undergo 3-yearly colonoscopic screening from the age of 35 years.

The role of the clinical geneticist

High-risk families

The clinical geneticist and genetic counsellors are particularly involved with the management of families at high risk of developing cancer. The genetics unit as a whole has a part to play in recommending management strategies for those at moderate or population risk of developing cancer via a strategy such as the West Midlands Family Cancer Strategy (WMFACS), where information about family histories is collected by family history questionnaire as described in Figure 3.8.

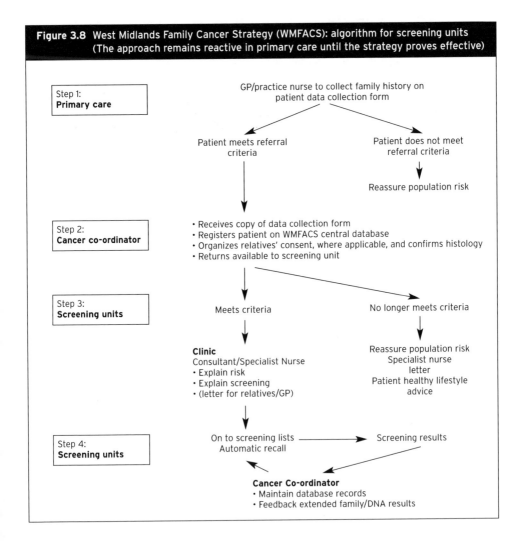

Figure 3.8 West Midlands Family Cancer Strategy (WMFACS): algorithm for screening units (The approach remains reactive in primary care until the strategy proves effective)

Step 1:
Primary care

GP/practice nurse to collect family history on patient data collection form

Patient meets referral criteria

Patient does not meet referral criteria

Reassure population risk

Step 2:
Cancer co-ordinator

- Receives copy of data collection form
- Registers patient on WMFACS central database
- Organizes relatives' consent, where applicable, and confirms histology
- Returns available to screening unit

Step 3:
Screening units

Meets criteria

No longer meets criteria

Clinic
Consultant/Specialist Nurse
- Explain risk
- Explain screening
- (letter for relatives/GP)

Reassure population risk
Specialist nurse letter
Patient healthy lifestyle advice

Step 4:
Screening units

On to screening lists
Automatic recall

Screening results

Cancer Co-ordinator
- Maintain database records
- Feedback extended family/DNA results

The geneticist is concerned with the identification of families at high risk of developing colorectal or other associated cancers (such as in HNPCC). Following the high-risk arm of the WMFACS model discussions, confirmation and extension of family history will take place and recommendations about colonic and gynaecological surveillance, dependent on family history, will be made. If the family history is significant, there may be a possibility of undertaking genetic testing. For this to be undertaken, DNA (usually from a blood sample) needs to be obtained (unless previously stored) from an affected family member. Before an affected family member provides blood for diagnostic DNA analysis, he or she will need to be seen in order to discuss the implications of undergoing genetic testing, including the following:

- Psychological issues such as the anxiety and worry created by undergoing mutation analysis, and the implications for the family. This may be particularly the case if the family history referral has been instigated by another family member (such as a niece or nephew). It is important to ensure that the individual does not feel under pressure to provide a blood sample for analysis.
- If the mutation analysis reveals a genetic fault (such as a *MLH1*, *MSH2* or *MSH6* gene mutation), the affected individual is at increased risk of developing cancers such as endometrial, ovarian or stomach cancers, etc. If this is the case, regular surveillance will be offered. If a mutation is identified, predictive genetic testing may be offered to other family members.
- If a genetic fault is not found, this may mean that the family history of cancer is not caused by the known gene faults currently identifiable. However, in the future it may be possible to identify a family fault as genetic knowledge increases or as laboratory techniques become more sophisticated. In this case the DNA will be retested at a later date. Family members will be encouraged to continue routine surveillance because they will still be at increased risk.

Predictive testing

If a gene fault is identified in a family then other susceptible individuals in a family can be tested for the same genetic mutation. If a genetic fault is known and individuals decide not to determine whether they are gene carriers, surveillance will continue to be offered until such time as they are ready to have their DNA examined for the fault. If an individual is found not to carry the family genetic fault, their risk of developing colorectal cancer and other related cancers (such as in HNPCC) falls back to that of the population, and additional screening outside that of population programmes is not recommended.

The client should have several opportunities to discuss the implications of genetic testing before this is undertaken in order to determine whether he or she is prepared for the test. If an individual is going through a stressful period in life, such as moving house, taking exams, etc. the test can be delayed until he or she feels ready (if ever).

In addition, as there could be financial issues for the individual if he or she undertakes testing, it would seem sensible for the individual to have taken out relevant insurance policies, etc. before the test because, if the gene fault is found, this may make obtaining life/health insurance, etc. more difficult or expensive in the future. There are currently discussions occurring between the Government and insurance organizations about this issue.

The psychological implications of genetic testing and feelings that the client may experience, such as anxiety about cancer risk and worries about passing on the faulty gene to children, are discussed before testing. Genetic counselling may help the client to clarify his or her feelings and anxieties and rehearse coping strategies to deal with the test results.

Population-risk families

As cancer is so common, with one in three individuals having the disease, particularly as they get older, many individuals will report having a family history of cancer. As previously described, those at more than twice population risk should be referred through to the local genetics unit or family history service. Individuals at near population risk (Figure 3.9) can be reassured that, based on current evidence, regular colonoscopies outside national screening programmes are not recommended, and general healthy lifestyle advice given.

Surveillance

Colorectal cancer can be detected by a variety of methods, including:

- faecal occult blood testing
- digital examination of rectum
- rigid sigmoidosopy
- flexible sigmoidoscopy
- colonoscopy
- barium enema
- tumour markers (carcinoembryonic antigen or CEA).

High-risk groups

These include those with family histories of FAP and HNPCC, those

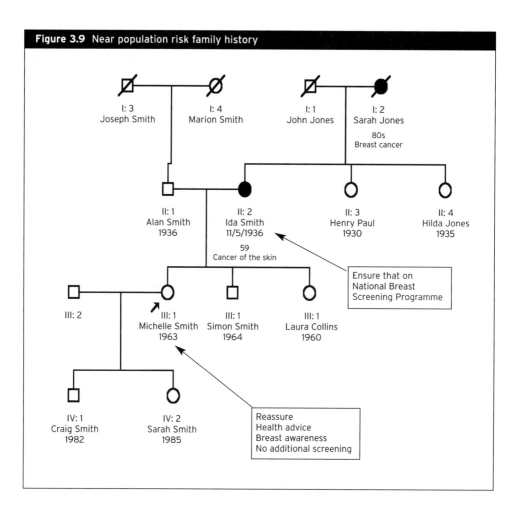

Figure 3.9 Near population risk family history

fulfilling the modified Amsterdam criteria and those just outside the guidelines with significant family histories.

Moderate-risk groups

COG guidelines suggest that people over the age of 50 with a first-degree relative should be offered FOB testing or flexible sigmoidoscopy.

Population risk groups

National trials are ongoing with regard to population screening, employing the methods of FOB testing and flexible sigmoidoscopy.

Symptomatic individuals

Symptomatic individuals should be referred to the appropriate fast track service as necessary. Those who are symptomatic and have family histories, should have their symptoms investigated first, and their family histories investigated separately.

Why screen for colorectal cancer?

Most colorectal cancer occurs as a result of a malignant change in adenomas that have occurred in the bowel lining 10–15 years earlier. Scholfield (2001) suggests that only 10 per cent of 1-cm adenomas become malignant after 10 years. In the general population the incidence of adenomatous polyps increases with age. Adenomatous polyps can be found in 20 per cent of the population, but 95 per cent are unlikely to become cancerous.

There is a known premalignant (adenoma) stage and there is a relatively long transitional stage from adenoma to carcinoma formation. As described in Chapter 2, a 1-cm lesion will take about 2–3 years to develop and about 7–10 years to develop into a carcinoma. As there is a long preclinical phase, there is a potential for early detection by screening asymptomatic individuals and therapeutic intervention is usually possible. Atkin (2002) states that most early adenomas and cancers are usually asymptomatic. A population screening plan could thus potentially reduce mortality from the disease. Selby et al. (1992) report that screening sigmoidoscopy reduces the risk of developing colorectal cancer, and there have been several studies illustrating this point by using FOB testing.

Population screening demands that screening tests are:

- inexpensive
- reliable
- acceptable
- specific and sensitive.

The WHO guidelines further suggest that the long-term benefits should outweigh the disadvantages. The screening test should be simple, and adequate compliance rates can be achieved.

Thus, when discussing methods of population screening, digital rectal examination and rigid sigmoidoscopy have limitations because patients may find these procedures unpleasant. Furthermore, they are invasive and may be limited because the whole bowel is not examined, so potentially some cancers may be missed.

Digital rectal examination

Only 10–15 per cent of cases of colorectal cancer are found using this approach. It may be useful as a baseline investigation and is often combined with flexible sigmoidoscopy.

Faecal occult blood tests

This investigation aims to detect early asymptomatic cancers and is based on the premiss that such cancers will bleed and small quantities of blood will be detectable chemically or immunologically in the stool. This is a simple and cheap investigation; however, Hobbs (2001) recommends that the low specificity of the test results in 40 per cent of cancers and 80 per cent of adenomas being missed. In addition, false positives result in 1–3 per cent requiring additional screening in the form of colonoscopy. False positives occur as a result of eating red meat, uncooked vegetables and fruit, drugs containing iron and non-steroidal anti-inflammatory medicines. Developments in immunological FOB tests may reduce this problem. As lesions tend to bleed later in their formation, this suggests that early cancers may be missed and there is a need for frequent testing. There may be about a 40 per cent occurrence of false negatives if FOB testing is used alone because tumour bleeding may not occur and/or may be intermittent. The sensitivity of the test requires that a 2 ml/day blood loss should be detectable.

The test most commonly used is based on guaiac (Haemoccult II) which needs a 20 ml blood loss per day to be detected. The test can be administered by collecting two samples from three consecutive stools and smeared on six cards. In the presence of blood the guaiac turns blue when exposed to hydrogen peroxide. From a variety of FOB testing trials (Hardcastle et al., 1996; Kronborg et al., 1996), Atkin (2002) suggests that annual FOB screening reduces the mortality from colorectal cancer by 33 per cent and biannual screening by 15–21 per cent. Further issues that may arise include the age of commencement of the test, because it may be that if individuals have started the test at 50 and have an unremarkable result (when the disease incidence is comparatively low), they may not see the necessity for continued testing. Other reasons for non-participation may include low socioeconomic status, being male, dietary restrictions before the test, being asymptomatic and not wanting to know about health problems (Atkin, 2002). There may also be the necessity to ensure that screen-positive patients continue forward for colonoscopic screening because this has been found to be a problem in the USA (Lurie and Welsh, 1999).

FOB testing appears to be promising as a tool for population screening in the over-50s, and early reports of high detection rates from 3-year trials in Coventry and Warwickshire and Fife, and Grampian and Tayside in Scotland, suggest that this may be adopted as a method of population screening. The test is being offered to 50–69-year-olds and results are expected to be available soon.

Flexible sigmoidoscopy

This procedure, using a 60-cm flexible sigmoidoscope, examines the whole of the left (sigmoid) colon and rectum, where 60 per cent of cancers are found. A major disadvantage is that 40 per cent of the colon is not examined, where 40 per cent of cancers and adenomas are detected.

A flexible sigmoidoscopy is more expensive then a rigid sigmoidoscopy and is generally more acceptable for patients because the procedure is more comfortable and requires no sedation. Scholfield (2001) recommends that adults should have a single colonoscopy undertaken between the ages of 55 and 65 to detect polyps; however, there are questions about the cost-effectiveness of this approach. Indeed, in the USA this procedure is routinely undertaken for all adults over 40 on a 3- to 5-yearly basis in this age range. There is an ongoing multicentre national trial evaluating the benefit of a single colonoscopy at 55 as a method of population screening.

As many nurses are now trained to undertake flexible sigmoidoscopy, the use of this as a potential screening tool is more feasible and cost-effective. Patient uptake has been estimated at 45 per cent and potentially 6 per cent will require full colonoscopy. Although the procedure may be initially expensive there are significant advantages over FOB testing because it is highly effective as a method of detecting adenomas and such polyps may be removed at the time of the procedure with no follow-up needed.

Winawer et al. (1987) suggest that development from adenomas to cancer takes about 10 years and therefore Atkin (2002) argues that the screening can be undertaken less frequently, depending on the age when it is initially undertaken. Evidence that sigmoidoscopy reduces rates of colorectal cancer have been demonstrated by a variety of studies; in one study the chance of developing distal colorectal cancer was reduced by 60 per cent in those undergoing flexible sigmoidoscopy (Selby et al., 1992). Other studies highlight that it is the detection and removal of adenomatous polyps that reduce the risk of colorectal cancer (Muller and Sonnenberg, 1995). Kavanagh et al. (1998) state that there is no advantage of colonoscopy over sigmoidoscopy in reducing the incidence of colorectal cancer.

However, there are suggestions that the procedure requires extensive staff training, causes discomfort, is time-consuming and invasive, and perforation can occur (although this is much lower than for colonoscopy), and bowel preparation is required. However, often only a single patient-administered enema is required and thus it is much less extensive than preparation for bowel colonoscopy (Scholfield, 2001). There may be issues with compliance and levels of only 45–49 per cent have been reported, which may be due to factors similar to those of non-compliance with FOB testing. Levels of compliance for colonoscopy are, however, lower than for flexible sigmoidoscopy. Interestingly, Atkin (2002) reports studies with higher levels of attendance among men than among women.

Ongoing trials into the efficacy of flexible sigmoidoscopy are continuing, including a UK and Italian trial examining efficacy of a single flexible sigmoidoscopy and the utility of adenoma removal (Atkin et al., 2001). The USA trial PLCO (prostate, lung colon and ovary) aims to examine the effect of colonic screening and screening for other cancers; it started in 1994 (Prorok et al., 2000). Results from the UK and Italian trials have been encouraging in that there was a significant uptake rate – 71 per cent of those invited for screening attended. The expected rate of individuals requiring follow-on colonoscopies after flexible sigmoidoscopy were in the region of 5 per cent, with ongoing analysis of the effects of screening for and removal of distal colorectal adenomas on colorectal occurrence and mortality rates. Atkin (2002) argues that before this could be used as a population screening tool there would need to be substantial investment in training and facilities available for endoscopic surveillance. The long waiting lists and lack of adequately trained endoscopists may be to blame for the lower survival rates for colorectal cancer in the UK compared with other countries (Gatta et al., 2000).

Colonoscopy

This procedure would not be acceptable as a population screening tool because of the need for full bowel preparation and sedation, making the procedure expensive, invasive and inconvenient. In addition there is a risk of bowel perforation, in the region of 1 in 6000. This is the procedure of choice for high-risk patients or those with a family history. This is because patients with family histories are more likely to develop polyps on the right side of their colon.

Colonoscopy enables the endoscopist potentially to see the whole of the mucosal lining of the colon and to remove small polyps in one session. Limitations include the inability to examine the bowel fully owing to failed bowel preparation and/or not being able to visualize the caecum. Errors may occur in the localization of tumours, owing to the lack of definite landmarks and difficulty in reaching and identifying the ileocaecal valve. As there are blind spots in the colon, the inexperienced colonoscopist may potentially miss large lesions, especially in the rectal ampulla and caecum, and around the acute bends. There is also the possibility of over- or under-sedation of patients, leading to pain and discomfort. Patients may be anxious and fearful about the procedure and find the bowel preparation unpleasant; this may lead to non-compliance or non-attendance. In addition patients may find the procedure embarrassing or distasteful. Perhaps if there is a real fear of the procedure, virtual colonoscopy in the form of computed tomography (CT) may be a possibility.

Management of polyps

If polyps are identified, these should be evaluated in terms of size, type and position, e.g. if they are pedunculated, sessile, elevated or flat with areas of depression. Sessile or flat polyps with or without areas of depression may be potentially early carcinoma. Management of early cancers may be undertaken by colonoscopic polypectomy for pedunculated adenomas, with focal carcinoma not undertaking the stalk. For early or focal carcinomas, annual colonoscopy is recommended until there have been two consecutive years without polyps, after which a 3-yearly surveillance colonoscopy is recommended.

Barium enema

This procedure has a role in confirming suspected lesions identified on colonoscopy. However, barium enema requires bowel preparation, and is expensive and uncomfortable.

Barium enema is unsuitable as a population screening tool as a result of these factors, and also because there would be inadequate radiology services to support the demand. In addition, polyps and Dukes' A carcinoma may be difficult to detect using this method, and furthermore polyps cannot be removed and so a colonoscopy would also be required if these are identified. However, combined with a flexible sigmoidoscopy, barium enema can be a useful surveillance tool.

Double-contrast barium enema

This procedure is sometimes used as a screening tool but has low sensitivity for cancer and large polyps.

Tumour markers

Carcinogen embryonic antigen (CEA) can be measured in patients who may be at risk of colorectal cancer. However, this is an unreliable marker because increased levels of CEA have also been found in patients with stomach, laryngeal and lung cancer. Furthermore, increased levels have been found in patients with ulcerative colitis, Crohn's disease or diverticular disease. The lack of specificity would make it inappropriate to use as a screening tool. Other biomarkers that have been used are CA50, CA195 and CA125; however, sensitivity is more unreliable then CEA and they are unlikely to be used as screening techniques, although they may have a part to play in the prediction of tumour prognosis. Studies that have identified *k-ras* gene deletion in the stools of individuals with colon cancer may therefore be useful as a future screening tool.

Computed tomography: virtual colonoscopy

This procedure requires full bowel preparation but is minimally invasive. Scholfield (2001) suggests that views of the bowel can be obtained in under 5 minutes. However, it is not currently widely available as a screening tool.

Ultrasonography and magnetic resonance imaging are also occasionally used as bowel surveillance tools.

References

Atkin W, Edwards R, Wardle et al. (2001) Rationale and design of a multicentre randomised trial to evaluate the suitability of flexible sigmoidoscopy as a mass population screening tool to reduce colorectal cancer morbidity and mortality. Journal of Medical Screening 8(3): 137-44.

Atkin WSA (2002) Effectiveness of colorectal screening. In: Cunningham D, Topham C, Miles A (eds), The Effective Management of Colorectal Cancer, 2nd edn. London: Aesculapius Medical Press, pp. 55-68.

Baron JA, Gerhardsson de Verdier M, Ekbom A (1994) Coffee, tea, tobacco and cancer of the large bowel. Cancer Epidemiology, Biomarkers and Prevention 3: 565-570.

Bird CL, Swendseid ME, Witte JS et al. (1995) Red cell and plasma folate, folate consumption and the risk of colorectal adenomatous polyps. Cancer Epidemiology, Biomarkers and Prevention 4: 709-714.

Boyle P, Langman JS (2001) In: Kerr D, Young AM, Hobbs FDR (eds), ABC of Colorectal Cancer: London: BMJ Publishing Group.

Burlow S (1987) Familial adenomatous polyposis: Danish Medical Journal 34: 1-15.

Burn J, Chapman PD, Mathers J et al. (1995) The protocol for a European double blind trial and resistant starch in familial adenomatous polyposis: the CAPP study. European Journal of Cancer: 31A: 1385-1386.

Burt RW (2000) Colon cancer screening. Gastroenterology 119: 837-853.

Cancer Outcomes Guidance (1997) Improving Outcomes for Colorectal Cancer. London: NICE.

Chyou PH, Nomura AM, Stemmermann GN (1996) A prospective study of colon and rectal cancer amongst Hawaii Japanese men. Annals of Epidemiology 6: 276-282.

Cole TRP, Sleightolme HV (2000) ABC of colorectal cancer: the role of clinical genetics in management. British Medical Journal 321: 1779-1780.

Cole T, Weiner C, Sleightholme HV (2002) Cancer and genetics and colorectal cancer: understanding how current data should be influencing routine clinical practice. In: Cunningham D, Topham C, Miles A (eds), The Effective Management of Colorectal Cancer, 2nd edn. London: Aesculapius Medical Press, pp. 33-53.

Dunlop MG (2002) Guidance on gastrointestinal surveillance for hereditary, non-polyposis colorectal cancer, familial adenomatous polyposis, juvenile polyposis and Peutz-Jeghers syndrome. Gut 51(suppl 5): 21-27.

Emerson JC, Weiss NS (1992) Colorectal cancer and solar irradiation. Cancer Causes and Control 3: 95-99.

Farrington SM, Lin-Goerke J, Wang Y et al. (1998) Systematic analysis of mis-match repair genes in colon cancer patients and controls. American Journal of Human Genetics 63: 749-759.

Garland CF, Comstock GW, Garland GW et al. (1989) Serum 25-hydroxyvitamin D and colon cancer: eight year prospective study. Lancet ii: 1176-1178

Gatta G, Capaocaccia R, Sant M et al. (2000) Understanding variations in survival for colorectal cancer in Europe: a EUROCARE high resolution study. Gut 47: 533-538.

Giovannucci E, Rimm EB, Stampfer MJ, Colditz GA, Ascherio A, Willet WC (1994) Intake of fat, meat and fibre in relation to colon cancer risk in men. Cancer Research 54: 2390-2397.

Hardcastle J, Chamberlain J, Robinson M et al. (1996) Randomised controlled trial of faecal occult blood screening for colorectal cancer: Lancet 348: 1472-1477.

Hardy R (2002) Molecular bases for risk factors in colorectal cancer - genetic syndromes, adenomatous colorectal polyps and ulcerative colitis. In: Cunningham D, Topham C, Miles A (eds), The Effective Management of Colorectal Cancer, 2nd edn. London: Aesculapius Medical Press, pp. 13-32.

Hardy RG, Meltzer SJ, Jankowski A (2001) In: Kerr DJ, Young AM, Hobbs R (2001) ABC of Colorectal Cancer: London: BMJ Books

Hirota C, Iida M, Aoyagi K et al. (1996) Effect of indomethacin suppositories on rectal polyposis in patients with familial adenomatous polyposis. Cancer 78: 1660.

Hobbs FDR (2001) In: Cunningham D, Topham C, Miles A (eds), The Effective Management of Colorectal Cancer, 2nd edn. London: Aesculapius Medical Press.

Hodson SV, Maher ER (1999) A Practical Guide to Human Cancer Genetics, 2nd edn. Cambridge: Cambridge University Press:

Houlston RS, Murday V, Harocopos C, Williams CB, Slack J (1990) Screening and genetic counselling for relatives of patients with colorectal cancer in a family cancer clinic. British Medical Journal 301: 366-368.

Kavanagh A, Giovannucci E, Fuchs C, Colditz G (1998) Screening endoscopy and risk of colorectal cancer in united states men. Cancer Causes and Control 9: 455-462.

Kerr DJ, Young AM, Hobbs R (eds) (2001) ABC of Colorectal Cancer. London: BMJ Books.

Kronborg O, Fenger C, Olsen J et al. (1996) Randomised study of screening for colorectal cancer with faecal-occult-blood test. Lancet 348: 1467-1471.

Langman M, Boyle P (2002) Colorectal cancer epidemiology. In: Cunningham D, Topham C, Miles A (eds), The Effective Management of Colorectal Cancer, 2nd edn. London: Aesculapius Medical Press, pp. 3-12.

Lovett E (1976) Family studies in cancer of the colon and rectum. British Journal of Surgery 63: 13-18

Lurie J, Welsh H (1999) Diagnostic testing following fecal occult blood screening in the elderly. Journal of the National Cancer Institute 91: 1641.

Lynch HT, Smyrck TC, Watson P et al. (1993) Genetics, natural history, tumour spectrum and pathology of hereditary non-polyposis colorectal cancer: an updated review. Gastroenterology 104: 1535-1549.

Muller A, Sonnenberg A (1995) Prevention of colorectal cancer by flexible endoscopy and polypectomy. Annals of Internal Medicine 123: 904–910.

Newcomb BA, Storer BE (1995) Postmenopausal hormone use and risk of large bowel cancer. Journal of the National Cancer Institute 87: 1067–1071

Peleg I, Maibach HT, Brown SH et al. (1994) Aspirin and non-steroidal anti-inflammatory drug use and the risk of subsequent colorectal cancer. Archives of Internal Medicine 154: 394.

Prorok P, Andriole G, Bresalier R et al. (2000) Design of the Prostate, Lung, Colorectal and Ovarian (PLCO) cancer screening trial. Controlled Clinical Trials: 21(suppl 6): 273S–309S.

Saffrey J, Stewart M (1997) Maintaining the Whole. Milton Keynes: Open University.

Scholfield JH (2001) In: Kerr D, Young AM, Hobbs FDR (eds), ABC of Colorectal Cancer. London: BMJ Books.

Selby JV, Friedman GD, Quesenberry CJ, Weiss NS (1992) A case-control study of screening sigmoidoscopy and mortality from colorectal cancer: New England Journal of Medicine 653–657.

Skirton H, Patch C (2002) Genetics for Healthcare Professionals: A lifestage approach. Oxford: Bios Scientific Publishers

Syngal S, Fity EA, Eng C et al. (2000) Sensitivity and specificity of clinical criteria for hereditary non-polyposis colorectal cancer associated mutations in MSH2 and MLH1. Journal of Medical Genetics 37: 641–645

Vasen HAS, Wijnen JT, Menko FH et al. (1996) Cancer risk in families with hereditary non-polyposis colorectal cancer diagnosed by mutation analysis. Gastroenterology 110: 1020–1027.

Vasen HFA, van Ballegooijen M, Buskens E et al. (1998) A cost effective analysis of colorectal screening of hereditary non-polyposis gene carriers. Cancer 82: 1632–1637.

Vasen HFA, Griffioen G, Offerhaus GJA et al. (1990) The value of screening and central registration of families with familial adenomatous polyposis: A study of 82 families in the Netherlands: Diseases of the Colon and Rectum 33: 227–230.

Willetts WC, Stampfer MJ, Colditz GA, Rosner BA, Speizer FE (1990) Relation of meat, fat and fiber intake to the risk of colon cancer in a prospective study among women. New England Journal of Medicine 323: 1664–1672

Winawer S, Zauber AG, Diaz B, Workgroup NPS (1987) The National Polyp Study: temporal sequence of evolving colorectal cancer from the normal mucosa. Gastrointestinal Endoscopy 33: 167.

Useful website addresses

www.geneclinics.org
www.nih.gov
www.cancergenetics.org
www.cancerhelpuk.org
www.cancerbacup.org.uk
www.beatingbowelcancer.org
www.coloncancer.org.uk

Chapter 4
Diagnosis and investigations
Yvette Perston

In the UK 20–40 per cent of patients with bowel cancer are diagnosed with incurable disease and 20 per cent of patients are admitted as emergencies (Mella et al., 1997). Politically driven initiatives to achieve early diagnosis have been launched on the assumption that this will lead to earlier presentation and thus increased survival. Improved public awareness of the condition has been achieved by health care initiatives and involvement of voluntary organizations. As awareness of bowel cancer and the symptoms associated with this diagnosis are increasing, there has been a rise in demand for rapid access to diagnostic services. The White Paper *The New NHS* proposed the following standard:

> Everyone with suspected cancer will be able to see a specialist within 2 weeks of their GP deciding that they need to be seen urgently and requesting an appointment
>
> Department of Health (DoH, 1997)

Patients with a high probability of having cancer can be identified statistically by the combination and persistence of their symptoms. Diagnostic services would be overwhelmed if all patients with bowel symptoms were referred for hospital assessment. A responsive service would diagnose most cancers by identifying those at high risk, but most patients would still need to be assessed and followed up in primary care.

As a large proportion of the population experience bowel symptoms every year, it is important that those who develop new symptoms are observed in general practice. Only those with persistent, progressive or sinister symptoms should be referred for rapid diagnosis. This does not mean that those who experience symptoms should delay presentation to their GP. A major impediment to patients consulting is embarrassment and reluctance to discuss bowel function. It is hoped that continuing efforts by health care professionals and voluntary organizations will break down this prejudice.

It is important that those who undergo urgent hospital investigation have a symptom complex that is statistically likely to be the result of cancer. Not only does this use resources effectively, but it also prevents psychological and physical harm to patients who are unlikely to have serious disease. When initiating investigations the inherent risks should be borne in mind.

Guidelines based on single symptoms result in large numbers of patients being referred for investigations, and they should be developed to ensure that only those patients with symptoms associated with a high risk of colorectal cancer are seen within the 2-week rule (Association for Coloproctology of Great Britain and Ireland or ACPGB&I, 2002). This is achieved by using symptom combinations that show high sensitivity and specificity, i.e. they include most patients with cancer, while excluding the majority with benign disease. It is accepted that some patients will present with atypical disease and so will not fall into these categories.

Symptoms

The site of the tumour in the colon often determines clinical presentation. Right-sided or caecal lesions often present with iron deficiency anaemia, diarrhoea or a palpable mass in the right iliac fossa, but are less likely to present with intestinal obstruction unless the ileocaecal valve itself is involved. Alteration of bowel habit, spurious diarrhoea and intestinal obstruction are more typical of lesions on the left side of the colon (Ellis et al., 1999). Rectal carcinoma presents with bleeding, tenesmus and change in bowel habit. However, only 40 per cent of patients present with typical features (Keddie and Hargreaves, 1968). The distribution of cancers throughout the colon is shown in Figure 4.1. the differential diagnosis is given in Table 4.1

Table 4.1 Differential diagnosis for different symptoms

Rectal bleeding	Diarrhoea	Constipation
Haemorrhoids	Diverticular disease	Crohn's disease
Perianal fissure	Infective colitis	Benign stricture
Infective colitis	Inflammatory bowel disease	Drug-induced
Inflammatory bowel disease	Coeliac disease	Poor dietary intake
Diverticular disease		
Angiodysplasia		
Meckel's diverticulum		

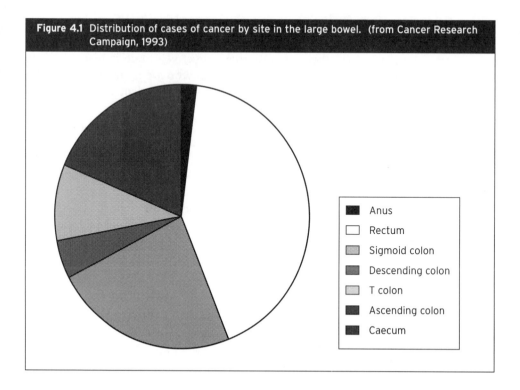

Figure 4.1 Distribution of cases of cancer by site in the large bowel. (from Cancer Research Campaign, 1993)

Legend:
- Anus
- Rectum
- Sigmoid colon
- Descending colon
- T colon
- Ascending colon
- Caecum

Rectal bleeding

A significant percentage of the community bleed every year (Fijten et al., 1994). Alone it has a low predictive value for colorectal cancer. The study of Thompson et al. (2000) found that only 1 in 709 patients with rectal bleeding in the community had cancer.

The colour of blood and its relationship to stool may give an indication of the site of the bleeding. Bright-red blood on the toilet paper or dripping after defecation is more commonly associated with an anal cause, e.g. haemorrhoids or fissures (Forde and Waye, 1989). Dark-red blood or blood mixed with the stool is more likely to be associated with colorectal cancer (Church, 1991), especially when associated with change in bowel habit and/or abdominal pain (Neugut et al., 1993). Rectal bleeding in cancer patients occurs without anal symptoms in over 60 per cent of patients (Dodds et al., 1999). The chance of these patients having cancer increases with age; Bat et al. (1992) reported a 29 per cent incidence of cancer in those aged over 80 years with rectal bleeding.

Alteration in bowel habit

It is important to appreciate that there is a wide range of defecatory frequency in the population. The normal range is from three times a day to once every three days. Consistency of stool varies with age, older patients having on average more formed stool, and also with gender, men on average having looser stools (Heaton et al., 1992a). Therefore, it is important to determine what has been normal for the individual and to assess whether any change warrants investigation.

A change in bowel habit is very common in the general population. Up to 30 per cent of individuals have an episode of constipation in any one year (Sonnenberg and Koch, 1989) and 6 per cent have an episode of diarrhoea persisting more than a few days (Dent et al., 1986).

It is important to ascertain exactly what patients mean by a change in bowel habit. Constipation is usually defined as the infrequent passage of hard stool with straining, whereas diarrhoea is the frequent passage of liquid or semi-liquid stool. Not only is consistency of stool important but also the frequency of defecation because change in frequency may be significant without a change in consistency.

Two hospital studies of cancer patients assessed the nature of the change in bowel habit and showed changes to looser stool and/or increased frequency in 87–91 per cent of patients with distal cancers and 61 per cent of patients with proximal cancers (Pescatori et al., 1982). Passage of mucus or excessive production of mucus can cause diarrhoea and may be the result of a carcinoma.

Pain

Abdominal pain is of surprisingly little help in assessing the likelihood of colorectal cancer because it is both very common in the population and large bowel obstruction tends to occur without warning. Abdominal pain is characterized by severity, timing and association with eating. With obstruction of the ileocaecal valve, intestinal colic may be experienced about an hour after eating when the bowel contents reach the caecum.

Abdominal pain is also a common symptom in the general population, 25–30 per cent of people suffering from it in any one year (Heaton et al., 1992b). It is also frequently associated with change in bowel habit, either constipation or diarrhoea.

Other significant symptoms suggesting rectal cancer are tenesmus and dyschezia. Tenesmus gives the feeling that a solid object is stuck in the anal canal, giving rise to a strong desire to defecate that cannot be satisfied. Dyschezia is a feeling that the rectum is still loaded with faeces after defecation.

Iron deficiency anaemia

A relatively small amount of ingested iron is absorbed in the upper intestinal tract. Occult gastrointestinal blood loss from colorectal cancer, particularly right-sided lesions, is an important cause of iron deficiency in men and postmenopausal women. In the age group where colorectal cancer is most prevalent, i.e. over 70 years, haemorrhoids or non-steroidal anti-inflammatory drugs should initially not be assumed to be the cause of iron deficiency anaemia and a full investigation should be undertaken. This would usually involve an upper gastrointestinal endoscopy but must include a colonoscopy or barium enema. All patients should undergo investigation of the lower gastrointestinal tract, even if an upper gastrointestinal pathology is diagnosed, because dual pathology is not uncommon (British Society of Gastroenterology, 2000).

Other presentations

Uncommon presentations occur in colorectal cancer as a result of advanced disease. Gastrocolic fistulae may cause faecal vomiting or severe diarrhoea and weight loss. Occasionally sigmoid cancers present as an external fistula or a psoas abscess. Internal fistulae can present with passage of faeces vaginally or recurrent urinary tract infections and pneumaturia. Local invasion of disease in rectal cancers produces localized pain and dysfunction.

Secondary dissemination of the disease may produce anorexia and weight loss. Occasionally patients present with distant metastases in the lung, brain or bone. These symptoms may be the only presenting features.

Emergency presentation

Admission as an emergency, often with advanced disease, is still common, being 20 per cent in the 1993 Welsh audit. Symptoms may have been present for only a short period of time and the patient usually presents with obstruction and/or perforation. Large bowel obstruction is characterized by lower abdominal pain, usually intermittent and colicky in nature, and absolute constipation. Increased bowel sounds (borborygmi), nausea, vomiting and distension usually accompany these.

A plain abdominal radiograph achieves confirmation of the diagnosis. This is often accompanied by a water-soluble contrast enema, because this can distinguish true obstruction from pseudo-obstruction or volvulus (Koruth et al., 1985).

Guidelines for referral

As discussed previously, bowel symptoms are very common in the general population and this has led to the development of guidelines for referral. The latest guidelines (ACPGB&I, 2002) have been developed to identify symptom combinations that maintain high sensitivity without loss of specificity and so include the majority of patients with cancer whilst excluding those with benign disease. However, this results in a few cancer patients with atypical presentations not being included in the category of urgent symptoms. Age is also an important factor in determining the risk of a patient having bowel cancer, as 85 per cent occur over the age of 60 years (Jolly et al., 1982).

These guidelines (Table 4.2) recommend the symptom combinations that should be used to identify patients who need referral under the 2-week standard.

Table 4.2 Guidelines for referral

	Age threshold
Rectal bleeding with change in bowel habit to looser stools and/or increased frequency persistent for 6 weeks	
Change in bowel habit as above WITHOUT rectal bleeding and persistent for 6 weeks	> 60 years
Rectal bleeding persistently WITHOUT anal symptoms	> 60 years
A definite palpable right-sided abdominal mass	All ages
A definite rectal mass (not pelvic)	All ages
Iron deficiency anaemia WITHOUT an obvious cause (<10g in postmenopausal women and <11g in men)	

Association for Coloproctology of Great Britain and Ireland (2002)

Outpatient assessment

Patients find talking about bowel symptoms embarrassing, so the practitioner should be perceptive to the sensitive nature of the subject and ensure privacy at all times. Many of the investigations undertaken to determine the diagnosis are invasive so it is vital to obtain fully informed consent. All stages of the consultation should be explained beforehand, including the reason for the procedure and any inherent risks.

A complete history should be taken to include presenting symptoms, past medical history, drug history and family history.

Blood tests should include full blood count, liver function tests and carcinoembryonic antigen (CEA). This is a tumour marker for colorectal cancer, but can be raised in other conditions, e.g. smokers (Lewis et al., 1984). It has limited use in diagnosis (Armitage, 1998).

Physical examination

General examination of the patient should look for evidence of weight loss, signs of general disease, jaundice, etc. Abdominal examination should be conducted with the patient supine and comfortable.

The examination should include:

1. Inspection: abdominal distension, visible peristalsis and scars indicating previous surgery.
2. Palpation: should include all four quadrants of the abdomen and inguinal regions, to elicit tenderness and detect abdominal masses. (May be able to feel palpable sigmoid colon; can be a normal finding in constipated patients.)
3. Percussion: dullness may suggest ascites or fluid-filled loops of bowel. Rebound tenderness indicates the presence of peritonitis.
4. Auscultation: listen for bowel sounds – high-pitched suggests partial obstruction; hypoactive bowel sounds may be present in late obstruction

Anorectal examination

This is traditionally performed in the left lateral position, but may be done in prone jack-knife, which can be embarrassing for the patient but often provides better views for the clinician. The anal area should be inspected, in good lighting, for rashes, lesions or skin tags.

A digital examination should be performed first. A gloved lubricated finger is placed flat on the anus, gentle pressure applied and when the sphincter yields the finger is passed into the anus. The suggested order of examination is to feel the rectum first, then extrarectal pelvic structures, the pelvic floor and finally the anal canal (Nicholls and Glass, 1985). The feel of mucosa and the anal canal should be smooth, so any masses are abnormal. An assessment of the pelvic floor relaxed and contracted should be made. The prostate in men and the cervix in women can be felt. Tenderness can indicate fissures or abscesses. The withdrawn finger should be inspected for stool, pus, mucus or blood. This examination is important, because there is a palpable mass in 40–80 per cent patients with rectal cancer (McSherry et al., 1969). On palpation, carcinoma is usually hard and ulcerated, often with everted edges. A vaginal examination should be carried out in women if there are associated gynaecological symptoms, e.g. vaginal discharge or dyspareunia.

Sigmoidoscopy

This is usually carried out after the digital examination. Many physicians prefer an unprepared bowel, as enemas can cause irritation that can mimic proctitis. It can also remove important physical signs such as mucus and blood and prevents inspection of stool. However, glycerine suppositories or a small-volume enema can be given if required.

It is usually performed in the left lateral position and can be with a rigid or flexible endoscope; the main advantage of the latter is the ability to insert beyond 20 cm.

The rigid scope is inserted with the obturator in place, initially in the direction of the umbilicus. When there is a fall in resistance (indicating that the rectum is entered) the obturator is removed and the instrument then angled along the sacrum. The instrument is advanced under direct vision with minimal insufflation, as far as possible or until the patient has discomfort. The instrument should be advanced only when the lumen ahead is visible. Inspection is performed during withdrawal, undertaking a circular motion so that all walls of the bowel are visualized. About 75 per cent tests will advance past the rectosigmoid junction (Nicholls and Glass, 1985) and it can be used to measure accurately distances from the anal verge, which may be important in deciding surgical options (Sands and Daniel, 1999).

Sigmoidoscopy allows close inspection of the mucosa for abnormalities, and the identification of blood or pus. It has a high specificity and sensitivity for polyps and cancers, but only in the left side of the colon. Sigmoidoscopy allows biopsy and snare excision of polyps. The risk of perforation with sigmoidoscopy is low (Gilbertson, 1974) and haemorrhage is a rare complication of biopsy.

Flexible sigmoidoscopy

This allows examination up to 60 cm and can usually be performed without sedation. Bowel preparation with a phosphate enema is usually sufficient, 1–2 hours before the test. Antibiotic prophylaxis is recommended for those patients at risk of developing endocarditis, e.g. those with prosthetic heart valves (Rex and Lewis, 1996).

The scope is usually inserted with the right hand and the controls manoeuvred in the left hand. The bowel is insufflated with air.

Examination of the mucosa is made on withdrawal of the instrument, the tip of the sigmoidoscope being rotated to cover all walls of the bowel. The yield of pathological abnormalities is greater than with rigid sigmoidoscopy; about 50 per cent of colorectal carcinomas are within reach of a flexible sigmoidoscope (Eddy et al., 1987). It provides a clearer visualization of the mucosa of the bowel and also tends to be more comfortable for the patient. Both biopsies and polypectomies can be performed using electrocautery.

Perforation rates are 1–2 per 10 000 (Winawer et al., 1997), being slightly higher when biopsy or polypectomy is performed. The position of the scope can be difficult to distinguish within the left colon, so the examination may be incomplete and assessments of tumour position may be inaccurate (Adam et al., 2000).

Further investigations

Faecal occult blood test

This test is often used in patients with unexplained iron deficiency anaemia. It is sensitive but not highly specific for colorectal cancer because it identifies any bleeding in the gastrointestinal tract, e.g. from gum disease or gastritis. About two-thirds of colorectal cancers bleed in the course of a week (Young and St John, 1991). However, bleeding is intermittent and may be missed using one-off tests. The test involves the patient adhering to a special diet, and restricting the use of anti-inflammatory drugs. It has been suggested (Leicester, 2000) that all patients with a positive faecal occult blood (FOB) test should have a colonoscopy, particularly as barium enemas can miss early lesions.

Colonoscopy

Resources for colonoscopy are still limited; a survey in 1997 indicated that less than 50 per cent of units were able to offer an adequate service (MacFarlane et al., 1999). Bowel preparation is usually sodium picosulphate given the day before the procedure. Sedation is generally given intravenously during the procedure, often with an antispasmodic or by pain relief. The technique can produce hypoxia, so oxygen saturation is monitored throughout with pulse oximetry.

The colonoscope is advanced under direct vision to the caecum; insufflation is with carbon dioxide or air. Careful examination is performed during withdrawal. The procedure should follow British Society of Gastroenterology guidelines (Bell et al., 1991).

Colonoscopy allows complete examination of the colon, and has a sensitivity and specificity of > 95 per cent for all lesions (Winawer et al., 1997). The major advantage of colonoscopy is greater sensitivity for small polyps and also that it allows tissue diagnosis and treatment when appropriate (Schofield et al., 1993).

The greatest risks of the procedure are perforation, which occurs in 1 in 1000, and haemorrhage, 3 in 1000; complication rates may be higher when a polypectomy is performed. About 2 in 10 000 will die as a result of the procedure (Waye et al., 1992). There are also worries about the completeness of the procedure; the Trent Wales audit (1993; Mella et al., 1997) reported completion rates as low as 50 per cent. Improved effectiveness of colonoscopy can be achieved with practice (Church, 1994), sedation (Rodney et al., 1993) and adequate bowel preparation (Church, 1994). A colonoscopy is known to be complete only when the ileocaecal valve is identified or a biopsy of the terminal ileum is retrieved (Cotton and Williams, 1990). The position of a tumour seen on colonoscopy is difficult to determine with accuracy as a result of the lack of landmarks (Cotton and Williams, 1990). A means of improving this is to use electromagnetic imaging (EMI). This is a method of imaging the three-dimensional position of the endoscope within the abdomen using a specially designed operating table (Saunders et al., 1995).

A recent development is the advent of nurses performing colorectal endoscopy. (Maule, 1994). The BSG have issued a document on the nurse endoscopist advising on training and supervision. The Joint Advisory Group (JAG, 1999) has identified minimum standards for units training in endoscopy – nurses are expected to train to the same standard as medics. There are now several nationally recognized nurse endoscopy training units.

Radiology

Any radiological investigation of the lower gastrointestinal tract should be considered only after full rectal examination including sigmoidoscopy.

Single contrast barium enema
This is a rarely performed procedure that does not involve insufflation of gas; it is less sensitive and specific than a double-contrast barium enema.

Double-contrast barium enema
This is the current radiological gold standard for examining the colon. Excellent bowel preparation is essential. This is usually achieved with a low residue diet and sodium picosulphate 24 hours before the procedure.

It is important to maintain an intake of at least 2 litres of clear fluids to avoid dehydration. During the procedure barium liquid is introduced through a balloon catheter placed in the rectum, the patient or table is rotated to coat all walls of the bowel, and most of the barium is removed. Insufflation of air or carbon dioxide through the catheter then enables an outline of the mucosa to be achieved. An antispasmodic may be given during the procedure because instillation of air may cause some discomfort. Using carbon dioxide instead of air as an insufflation gas reduces pain (Bloomfield, 1981). Patients continue to pass barium for 1–2 days after the test and may need laxatives to prevent constipation. This procedure is increasingly performed by radiographers, the resulting films being checked by consultant radiologists to reduce interpretation errors.

Barium enema has a sensitivity and specificity of over 80 per cent in diagnosing colorectal cancers (Winawer et al., 1997). Insensitivity is related to inadequate visualization of parts of the bowel as a result of excessive looping or errors of interpretation. False positives are mainly caused by retained stool and other mucosal irregularities. It is a safe test, complication rates being approximately 3 per 10 000 tests. Perforation occurs in 1 in 25 000 procedures (Gelfand et al., 1979). The technique should be avoided for 5 days after biopsy of the rectum (Harned et al., 1982).

There is some evidence to suggest that the earlier lesions are more likely to be missed. Farrands et al. (1983) reported that flexible sigmoidoscopy detected seven Dukes' A carcinomas out of eight tumours missed on barium enema. Rex et al. (1997) found 25 per cent Dukes' A lesions detected by colonoscopy compared with 10 per cent by barium enema.

Colorectal cancer usually appears as an irregular polypoid lesion or 'apple core' stricture (Figure 4.2). It is ideal to obtain a histological diagnosis, especially if a stoma is to be constructed. However, if the image is unequivocal and right sided, it is reasonable to continue with the treatment plan. The sigmoid colon can be difficult to examine, particularly in the presence of diverticular disease (Leicester, 2000). The rectum should always be visualized endoscopically because it is not outlined well with barium, and lesions may be missed (Reeders et al., 1995). However, a barium enema may be better at demonstrating fistulating disease.

All patients who have had a colorectal malignancy diagnosed should have the rest of the colon visualized preoperatively because the incidence of synchronous tumours is about 5 per cent (Finan et al., 1987). If not possible as a result of a stenosing lesion, it is recommended that it should be done within three months of surgery (Association for Coloproctology of Great Britain and Ireland, 2001).

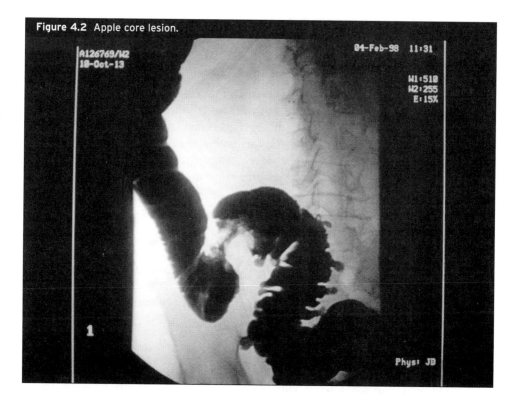

Figure 4.2 Apple core lesion.

Colonography/virtual colonoscopy

This is a relatively new procedure using spiral computed tomography (CT). This involves an X-ray tube that rotates continuously around the patient as he or she moves forwards on a table. This can produce three-dimensional images of the abdomen. Scan data are computed to produce images of the colon in three dimensions, similar to those obtained during a real colonoscopy. Patients have bowel preparation 24 hours before the test but do not need to be sedated. Intravenous smooth muscle relaxants are administered and the colon is insufflated with air through a rectal tube; then multiple cross-sectional scans are taken with the patient in both the supine and prone position to redistribute intraluminal fluid and enable adequate distension (Halligan and Fenlon, 1999). There may need to be simultaneous intravenous injection of contrast medium. The procedure takes only one minute. This technique is generally known as a CT pneumocolon. A computer constructs a three-dimensional endoluminal image of the whole colon, which the radiologist can view as a 'fly through' (Vining et al., 1994). The procedure can detect lesions larger than 1 cm with accuracy comparable to that of colonoscopy (Hara et al., 1997). It can give cross-sectional and endoluminal images and so can visualize lymph nodes and liver involvement in one examination. It can also be used preoperatively to image the entire colon in patients with obstructive disease. It may be the imaging technique of choice for elderly and frail patients who would not tolerate colonoscopy or barium enema, or for those in whom it is difficult to image the proximal right colon (Morrin et al., 2000). However, this technique is unable to provide a tissue diagnosis. This remains a developing procedure and as yet there are few large studies of its accuracy and effectiveness.

For staging

Staging schemes are designed to convey the anatomical extent of cancer within the body. Staging is important because it indicates the extent of the disease, and therefore the prognosis and likely outcome. Staging can be clinical, based on examination and investigations, or pathological, based on microscopic examination of the removed specimen. Usually, the stage of colorectal cancer can be defined accurately only after resection.

Two pathological staging systems are described in colorectal cancer. The first was the Dukes' classification (1930), originally to stage rectal cancer. This was further adapted in 1935 to subdivide stage C (Gabriel et al. 1945), and in 1945 (Dukes, 1945) when it became applied to colonic carcinoma (Table 4.3).

Table 4.3 Dukes' classification system

Stage A	Invasion not beyond the muscularis propria, no lymph node metastases
Stage B	Invasion beyond the muscularis propria, no lymph node metastases
Stage C1	Regional lymph node metastasis, without apical node involvement
Stage C2	Regional lymph node metastasis, without apical node involvement
(Stage D	Distant metastases – described by Turnbull et al. (1967)

The TNM system was developed as a system applicable to all tumour sites (UICC, 1966), being finally adopted internationally in 1992. A suffix is used in front of the stage to designate clinical (cTNM) and pathological (pTNM) (Table 4.4 and Figure 4.3).

Table 4.4 TNM clinical classification

T	Primary tumour
Tx	Primary tumour cannot be assessed
T0	No evidence of primary tumour
T1	Tumour invades submucosa
T2	Tumour invades muscularis propria
T3	Tumour invades through muscularis propria into subserosa or into non-peritonealized pericolic or perirectal tissues
T4	Tumour directly invades other organs or structures and/or perforates visceral peritoneum
N	Regional lymph nodes
Nx	Regional lymph nodes cannot be assessed
N0	No regional lymph node metastases
N1	Metastasis in one to three pericolic or perirectal lymph nodes
N2	Metastasis in four or more pericolic or perirectal lymph nodes
N3	Metastases in any lymph node along the course of a named vascular trunk
M	Distant metastases
Mx	Presence of distant metastases cannot be assessed
M0	No distant metastases
M1	Distant metastases

Residual tumour classification

Rx	Presence of residual tumour cannot be assessed
R0	No residual tumour
R1	Microscopic residual tumour
R2	Macroscopic residual tumour

International Union Against Cancer (UICC, 1992)

The circumferential resection margin is defined as the outer edge of the resected specimen of bowel and is particularly important in rectal cancer and total mesorectal excision (TME) surgery.

Quirke et al. (1986) demonstrated that the involvement of the circumferential resection margin in rectal cancer was an important predictor of local recurrence. Pathologists have now widely adopted his method of pathological examination to determine this risk in all rectal cancer patients.

Accurate staging of the disease allows an appropriate treatment plan to be devised for each individual patient. It is imperative that patients understand the importance of pre-treatment planning because it could be perceived that definitive treatment is being delayed by unnecessary tests.

Staging of colorectal cancer involves assessing the local extent and distant spread of the disease. About 20 per cent patients with newly diagnosed colorectal cancer will have metastatic disease. If definitive

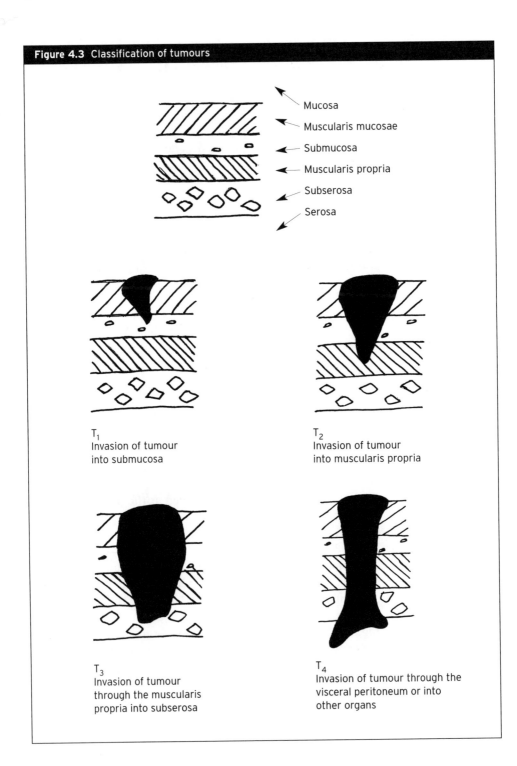

Figure 4.3 Classification of tumours

Mucosa
Muscularis mucosae
Submucosa
Muscularis propria
Subserosa
Serosa

T_1
Invasion of tumour
into submucosa

T_2
Invasion of tumour
into muscularis propria

T_3
Invasion of tumour
through the muscularis
propria into subserosa

T_4
Invasion of tumour through the
visceral peritoneum or into
other organs

treatment is started before staging is complete the patient may have inappropriate treatment, e.g. patients with multiple distant metastases may not need a bowel resection because their life expectancy is short and the symptoms from the primary may be minimal. Guidelines recommend that all patients, particularly those with rectal cancer, should have preoperative staging (Royal College of Surgeons, 1996; ACPGB&I, 2001).

Staging involves assessment of local and distant extent of the disease, so these are discussed separately.

Local staging of rectal cancer

Involvement of the circumferential resection margin (CRM), i.e. clearance of the cancer by less than 1 mm, is a predictor of local recurrence in rectal cancer (Quirke et al., 1986). One method of reducing local recurrence is to give preoperative chemo-/radiotherapy. Therefore, it is important to assess the local extent of disease in rectal cancer because this determines the suitability for preoperative treatment with radio-/chemotherapy and also the choice of surgical intervention from local excision to radical resection or sphincter-saving surgery.

Digital staging

Digitation of the tumour per rectum is the traditional method of clinical staging. A system was developed in the 1970s based on digital rectal examination alone. This method assesses local invasion of the rectal tumour by categorization of size, level and extent of tumour, and the degree to which it is fixed to the pelvis and surrounding structures. Nicholls et al. (1982) defined a system of four stages using this method (Table 4.5).

Table 4.5 Local extent assessed by digital examination

Stage 1	Confined to rectum
Stage 2	Confined to rectum or slight extrarectal spread
Stage 3	Moderate or extensive extrarectal spread
Stage 4	Involvement of other organs or unresectability

Nicholls et al. (1982)

Invasion within the rectal wall is difficult to identify, but gross spread can be accurately predicted in 80 per cent of cases. Understaging is a common problem and accuracy depends on the experience of the clinician. Fixation of the rectum is associated with a poorer prognosis (Nicholls et al., 1982), although it can result from local invasion or inflammation caused by the tumour (Durdey and Williams, 1984). Tumours of the middle or upper rectum may need to be examined under anaesthesia. The advantages of this method of staging are that it is inexpensive and freely available.

Endoanal ultrasonography

Patient preparation is two glycerine suppositories or an enema 1 hour before the test. Usually the patient is placed in jack-knife or left lateral position. The endorectal ultrasound probe is surrounded by a balloon filled with water and inserted into the rectum. It is advanced proximal to the tumour, the examination being performed during withdrawal. The difference in tissue density of the rectal wall produces a five-layer image that can be used to determine tumour invasion. Tumours are hypoechoic and, when invaded by tumour, the separate layers are distorted or disrupted. The accuracy for staging tumour penetration averages more than 80 per cent in published studies (Hildebrandt and Feifel, 1997). It is particularly useful in assessing the depth of penetration in early rectal tumours (Di Candio et al., 1987). Lymph nodes are visible when enlarged, their size being directly proportional to the risk of their containing metastatic disease; those smaller than 5 mm in diameter have a 20 per cent risk, whereas those larger than 9 mm have a 70 per cent risk (Heimann and Szporn, 1998). The accuracy of determination of mesorectal node involvement is only 50–60 per cent; this may be because many nodes lie outside the field of the probe (Glaser et al., 1990). The limitations of endoanal ultrasonography are its small field of view and inability to stage high or stenosing tumours. This prevents assessment of the CRM and prediction of surgical respectability. Some comparative studies show superiority of endorectal ultrasonography over CT and surface MRI in rectal cancer (Rifkin and Wechlser, 1986; Waizer et al., 1991).

This method of staging is used widely because it is relatively non-invasive and quick, and also widely available in most centres. As with most methods of staging, it is most accurate in assessment in expert hands (Glaser et al., 1990).

Computed tomography

Pelvic CT can be used to detect local spread of rectal cancer. Its accuracy depends on the thickness of the 'slices' and, as with all other methods, the experience of the operator. CT scans cannot distinguish the different layers of the rectal wall, and so are not able to distinguish between T_1 and T_2 tumours. Lymph nodes that appear enlarged are assumed to contain tumour deposits and CT can also identify extension beyond the bowel wall. However, as with endoanal ultrasonography it cannot be determined whether this is caused by invasion or inflammatory reaction. Various studies have reported accuracies of 50–80 per cent in comparison to histology (Angelelli et al., 1990). Thus, CT can predict resectability of the tumour with some accuracy. However, early tumours and those just invading through the wall cannot be assessed (Nicholls et al., 1982), and there is also wide variation in the accuracy of assessment of lymph nodes (Balthazar et al., 1988). For this reason CT is not widely used for assessment of rectal tumours.

Magnetic resonance imaging

This investigation uses the waveform of magnetic resonance of hydrogen nuclei in the body. This is picked up by a scanner and translated into visual images. Hydrogen nuclei are present in large numbers in fat and water, and so show up white. Organs show up in shades of grey. Movement produces blurring or motion artefact so it is vital that the patient stays still during the procedure. The tunnel effect and noise of the machine may cause claustrophobia so patients need to be well informed. There is a need to remove all clothing containing metal objects because they can cause artefacts. For the same reason, this examination cannot be used on patients with implanted metal objects, e.g. hip prostheses.

MRI is used in the assessment of spread of rectal cancer, with most studies finding sensitivity equal to that of CT (Hodgman, 1994; McNicholas et al., 1994). Enlarged nodes can be identified but there is difficulty distinguishing between inflammatory and neoplastic changes.

The use of an endorectal coil can enhance the image produced. This is inserted with the patient in the left lateral position and held there by use of a clamp to reduce motion artefact. This method provides detailed definition of primary tumour depth. However, they may be difficult to use in stenosing tumours and are more invasive. They are also less accurate in providing information about the circumferential resection margin because of the limited field of view (Zbar and Kmiot, 1998).

The most accurate current method is to use an external phased-array coil that provides images with high spatial resolution and also a wide field of view, allowing visualization of the entire mesorectum and surrounding pelvic organs (Beets-Tan et al., 2001). MRI can identify nodes of 2–3 mm in the mesorectum; those > 1 cm are likely to be involved (Brown et al., 1999). MRI is also able to predict whether the circumferential resection margin is likely to be threatened (Beets-Tan et al., 2001). MRI can accurately identify the lower edge of the tumour and so aid in the decision of whether sphincter-saving surgery is possible. It also allows prediction of the involvement of local organs e.g. seminal vesicles, vagina, and so allows planned modification of the surgical procedure to include their excision (Figure 4.4).

Figure 4.4 (a) Extension of tumour into bladder and into mesorectal fat. (b) Arrows show extramural invasion of tumour into the mesorectum.

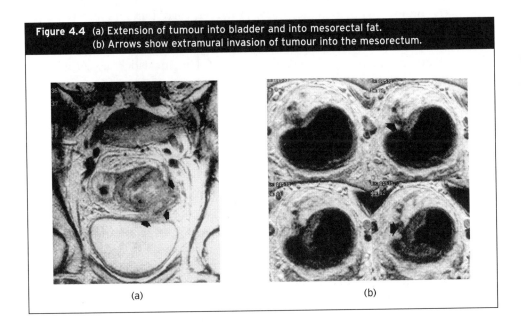

(a)   (b)

MRI is likely to increase in accuracy as technology improves, and is thus becoming the investigation of choice in local staging of rectal cancer.

Distant staging

This is performed to assess the distant spread of the disease. Colorectal cancer usually metastasizes to the liver and/or lungs, so these are the organs most commonly considered during investigation.

Chest radiograph

Up to 25 per cent of patients with distant spread will have pulmonary metastases. A plain chest radiograph will identify most pulmonary metastases, but a CT scan is more sensitive.

Ultrasonography

Ultrasound waves are produced by applying a short burst of electricity to a piezoelectric crystal in the transducer; several of these together comprise a probe. Diagnosis is made by measuring the echoes produced by the scattering of sound waves by the tissue interfaces. To scan a patient the probe is placed on the skin, gel being used to produce an air-free interface. To scan the liver a patient usually has to be nil by mouth for the day of the test because food can obstruct the scan preventing a clear view.

The sensitivity of ultrasonography in identifying liver metastases > 1 cm is 50–80 per cent (Heriot et al., 1999). Schreye et al. (1984) compared various methods of assessing liver metastases. Liver function tests had low sensitivity; ultrasonography and CT had an accuracy of 79–88 per cent with no significant difference between them. Ultrasonography is widely available and economical.

Intraoperative ultrasonography

Intraoperative ultrasonography can be performed either directly or laparoscopically and can obviate the need for preoperative CT as a staging procedure for distant metastases. This may be the most sensitive method for detecting liver metastases; Machi et al. (1987) reported an accuracy of 98 per cent for intraoperative ultrasonography in identifying liver metastases. Laparoscopy is also capable of detecting peritoneal deposits. It can be used at the time of surgery to determine whether a curative resection is possible. However, as yet it is not widely available and few studies have been done looking at its relative efficacy.

Computed tomography

Computed tomography provides a detailed liver and thorax image to stage distant disease (Figure 4.5). CT is accurate in detection of liver metastases > 1.5 cm in diameter (Levitt et al., 1977).

Positron emission tomography

Positron emission tomography (PET) with 2-fluoro-2-deoxy-D-glucose (FDG) is a whole-body imaging technique that exploits the increased rate of glycolysis in tumour cells to detect disease. Patients are fasted for four hours before the test, FDG is administered intravenously and a whole-body scan is undertaken. It is used principally to determine local or distant recurrence, especially when there is doubt about appearances on other imaging modalities. It is particularly useful in distinguishing cancer from inflammatory or scar tissue in postoperative patients. FDG PET

Figure 4.5 (a) CT scan showing liver metasteses.
(b) CT scan showing lung metasteses.

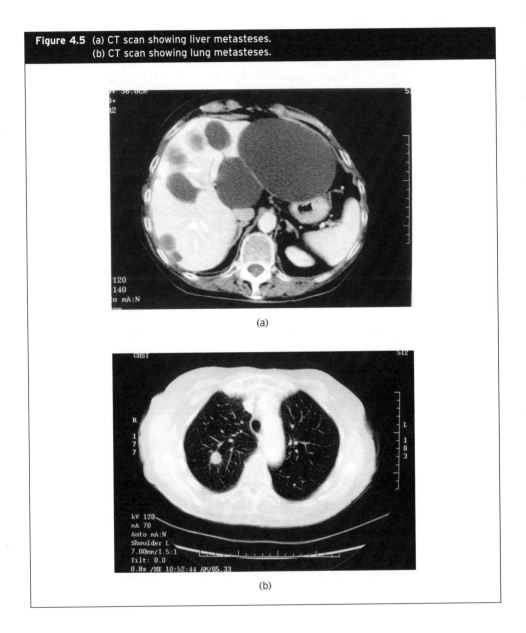

(a)

(b)

has been shown to be more accurate in the detection of total body tumour burden than a combination of other techniques, including CT and ultrasonography (Whiteford et al., 2000). However, it is very expensive and currently available only in major centres and therefore cannot be recommended for widespread use. Its main use is in the evaluation of patients who may benefit from curative hepatic resection, because it has an increased ability to detect additional hepatic disease compared with CT.

Radioimmunodetection

Colorectal tumours express carcinoembryonic antigen (CEA). Arcitumomab is an anti-CEA antibody labelled with technetium-99m. This can be given to the patient by intravenous infusion; imaging can then be carried out externally using a total body scan (radioimmunodetection or RAID). Alternatively a gamma probe can be used intraoperatively to identify any areas of tumour, e.g. in lymph nodes or locally invading other tissues (Hughes et al., 1997). Usually designated as RIGS (radioimmuno-guided surgery) this allows more predictive surgical resection to clear any areas of tumour involvement and allows surgeons the possibility of clearing metastatic disease. This technique is not yet widely available and is currently used only as part of research trials.

The multidisciplinary team in treatment planning

The concept of multidisciplinary teams (MDT) was first muted in the Calman–Hine report (Expert Advisory Group on Cancer, 1995). The aim was to unite a group of professionals who were all involved in caring for and treating cancer patients. This concept has since been developed nationally, and most hospitals now have active colorectal cancer MDTs that meet on a regular basis to discuss individual patients' treatment plans. The team usually consists of core members – the colorectal surgeon, pathologist, radiologist, oncologist and specialist nurse. Many have extended to include associate members such as the gastroenterologist and the palliative care team. The regular meeting of this group is the ideal place in which to discuss the diagnosis and staging of each patient (particularly those with rectal cancer) and to decide collectively on an appropriate treatment plan. All MDTs aim to treat patients in line with evidence-based national protocols, although patient choice may influence some treatment decisions. The MDT provides an ideal arena for audit of patient outcomes, thus enabling adaptation of management protocols with improving knowledge and providing a perfect platform for clinical governance issues.

References

Adam IJ, Ali Z, Shorthouse AJ (2000) How accurate is the endoscopist's assessment of visualisation of the left colon seen at flexible sigmoidoscopy? Colorectal Disease 2: 41-44.

Angelelli G, Scopinaro G, Claudiani F, Davini D, Mallarini G, Saitta S (1990) Rectal carcinoma: CT staging with water as a contrast medium. Radiology 177: 511-514.

Association of Coloproctology of Great Britain and Ireland (2001) Guidelines for the Management of Colorectal Cancer. London: Royal College of Surgeons.

Association of Coloproctology of Great Britain and Ireland (2002) Referral Guidelines for Bowel Cancer. London: Royal College of Surgeons.

Armitage, N (1998) Colorectal cancer: clinical features and investigations. Medicine 26: 975-976.

Balthazar EJ, Megibow AJ, Hulnick D, Naidich DP (1988) Carcinoma of the colon: detection and preoperative staging by CT. Radiology 150: 301-306.

Bat L, Pines A, Shemesh E et al. (1992) Colonoscopy in patients aged 80 years or older and its contribution to the evaluation of rectal bleeding. Postgraduate Medical Journal 68: 355-358.

Beets-Tan RGH, Beets GL, Vliegen RFA et al. (2001) Accuracy of magnetic resonance imaging in prediction of tumour-free resection margin in rectal cancer surgery. The Lancet 357: 497-504.

Bell GD, McCloy RF, Charlton JE et al. (1991) Recommendations for standards of sedation and patient monitoring during gastrointestinal endoscopy. Gut 32: 823-827.

Bloomfield JA (1981) Reliability of barium enema in detecting colonic neoplasia. Medical Journal of Australia 1: 631-633.

Brown G, Richards CJ, Newcombe RG et al. (1999) Rectal carcinoma: thin section MR imaging for staging in 28 patients. Radiology 211: 215-2222.

British Society of Gastroenterology (2000) Guidelines for the management of iron deficiency anaemia. Gut 46(suppl IV): 1-5.

Cancer Research Campaign (1993) Cancer of the Large Bowel Factsheet 18. London: CRC.

Church JM (1991) Analysis of the colonoscopic findings in patients with rectal bleeding according to the pattern of their presenting symptoms. Diseases of the Colon and Rectum 34: 391-395.

Church J (1994) Complete colonoscopy: how often? And if not, why not? American Journal of Gastroenterology 89: 556-560.

Cotton PB, Williams CB (1990) Practical Gastrointestinal Endoscopy, 3rd edn. Oxford: Blackwell Scientific Publications.

Dent OF, Goulston KJ, Zubrzychi J, Chapuis PH (1986) Bowel symptoms in an apparently well population. Diseases of the Colon and Rectum 29: 243-247.

Department of Health (1997) The New NHS - Modern, Dependable. London: Department of Health.

Di Candio G, Mosca F, Campatelli A, Cei A, Ferrari M, Basolo F (1987) Endosonographic staging of rectal carcinoma. Gastrointestinal Radiology 12: 289-295.

Dodds S, Dodds A, Vakis S et al. (1999) The value of various factors associated with rectal bleeding in the diagnosis of colorectal cancer. Gut 44: A99.

Dukes CE (1930) The spread of cancer of the rectum. British Journal of Surgery 17: 643-648.

Dukes CE (1945) Discussion on the pathology and treatment of carcinoma of the rectum. Proceedings of the Royal Society of Medicine 38: 381-384.

Durdey P, Williams NS (1984) The effect of malignant and inflammatory fixation of rectal carcinoma on prognosis after rectal excision. British Journal of Surgery 71: 787-790.

Eddy DM, Nugent FW, Eddy JF et al. (1987) Screening for colorectal cancer in a high-risk population. Gastroenterology 92: 682-92.

Ellis BG, Baig KM, Senpati A, Flashman K, Jaral M, Thompson MR (1999) Common modes of presentation of colorectal cancer patients. Colorectal Disease 1(suppl): 24.

Expert Advisory Group on Cancer to the Chief Medical Officers of England and Wales (1995) A Policy Framework for Commissioning Cancer Services. London: Department of Health.

Farrands PA, Vellacott KD, Amar SS, Balfour TW, Hardcastle JD (1983) Flexible fiberoptic sigmoidoscopy and double contrast barium enema examination in the identification of adenomas and carcinoma of the colon. Diseases of the Colon and Rectum 26: 725-727.

Fijten GH, Blijham GH, Knottnerus JA (1994) Occurrence and clinical significance of overt blood loss per rectum in the general population and in medical practice. British Journal of General Practice 44: 325.

Finan PJ, Ritchie JK, Hawley PR (1987) Synchronous and 'early' metachronous carcinomas of the colon and rectum. British Journal of Surgery 74: 945-994.

Forde KA, Waye JD (1989) Is there a need to perform full colonoscopies in a middle age person with episodic bright red blood per rectum and internal haemorrhoids? American Journal of Gastroenterology 84: 1227-1228.

Gabriel WB, Dukes CE, Bussey HJ (1945) Lymphatic spread in cancer of the rectum. British Journal of Surgery 23: 395-413.

Gelfand, DW, Ott DJ, Ramquist NA (1979) Pneumoperitoneum occurring during double-contrast enema. Gastrointestinal Radiology 4: 307-308.

Gilbertson VA (1974) Proctosigmoidoscopy and polypectomy in reducing the incidence of rectal cancer. Cancer 34: 936

Goulston KJ, Cook HI, Dent OF (1986) How important is rectal bleeding in the diagnosis of bowel cancer and polyps? The Lancet ii: 261-264.

Glaser F, Schlag P, Herfarth C (1990) Endorectal ultrasonography for the assessment of invasion of rectal tumours and lymph node involvement. British Journal of Surgery 77: 883-887.

Halligan S, Fenlon HM (1999) Virtual colonoscopy. British Medical Journal 319: 1249-1252.

Hara AK, Johnson CD, Reed JE et al. (1997) Detection of colorectal polyps with CT colonoscopy: initial assessment of sensitivity and specificity. Radiology 205: 59-65.

Harned RK Consigny, PM, Cooper, NB (1982) Barium enema examination following biopsy of the rectum or colon. Radiology 145: 11-16.

Heaton KW, Radvan J, Cripps H et al. (1992a) Defecation frequency and timing, and stool form in the general population; a prospective study. Gut 33: 529-534.

Heaton KW, O'Donnell LJD, Braddon FEM et al. (1992b) Symptoms of irritable bowel syndrome in a British urban community Gastroenterology 102: 1962-1967.

Heimann, TM, Szporn, AH (1998) Color Atlas of Preoperative Staging and Surgical Treatment Options in Rectal Cancer. Baltimore, Md: Williams & Wilkins.

Heriot AG, Grundy A, Kumar D (1999) Preoperative staging of rectal carcinoma. British Journal of Surgery 86: 17-28.

Hildebrandt U, Feifel G (1997) Preoperative staging: a critical analysis. Chapter in: Soreide O, Norstein J (eds) Rectal Cancer Surgery. Berlin: Springer-Verlag.

Hodgman CG, MacCarthy RL, Wolff BG et al. (1994) Preoperative staging of rectal carcinoma by computed tomography and 0.15T magnetic resonance imaging. Diseases of the Colon and Rectum 29: 446-450.

Hughes K, Pinsky CM, Petrelli NJ et al. (1997) Use of the carcinoembryonic antigen radio-immunodetection and computed tomography for predicting the respectability of recurrent colorectal cancer. Annals of Surgery 226: 621-631.

Joint Advisory Group (1999) Recommendations for Training in Gastrointestinal Endoscopy. London: Royal College of Physicians.

Jolly KD, Scott JP, MacKinnon MJ, Clarke AM (1982) Diagnosis and survival in carcinoma of the large bowel. Australia and New Zealand Journal of Surgery 52: 12-16.

Keddie N, Hargreaves A (1968) Symptoms of carcinoma of the colon and rectum. The Lancet ii: 749-750.

Koruth NM, Koruth A, Matheson MA (1985) The place of contrast enema in the management of large bowel obstruction. Journal of the Royal College of Surgeons of Edinburgh 30: 258-260.

Leicester RJ (2000) Colonoscopy - trials, triumphs and tribulations. In: Scholefield JH (ed.), Challenges in Colorectal Cancer. Oxford: Blackwell Science, pp. 105-125.

Levitt RG, Dagel SS, Stanley RJ, Jost RG. (1977) Accuracy of computed tomography of the liver and biliary tract. Radiology 124: 123-128.

Lewis H, Blumgart LH, Carter DC et al. (1984) Preoperative carcinoembryonic antigens and survivals in patients with colorectal cancer. British Journal of Surgery 71: 206-208.

Machi J, Isomoto H, Yamashita Y, Kurohiji T, Shirouzu K, Kakegawa T (1987) Intraoperative ultrasonography in screening for liver metastases from colorectal cancer: comparative accuracy with traditional procedures. Surgery 101: 678-684.

MacFarlane B, Leicester R, Romaya C, Epstein O (1999) Colonoscopy services in the United Kingdom. Endoscopy 31: 409-411.

McNicholas MMJ, Joyce WP, Dolan J et al. (1994) Magnetic resonance imaging of rectal carcinoma: a prospective study. British Journal of Surgery 81: 911-914.

McSherry CK, Cornell GN, Glenn F (1969) Carcinoma of the colon and rectum. Annals of Surgery 169: 502-509.

Maule W (1994) Screening for colorectal cancer by nurse endoscopists. New England Journal of Medicine 330: 183-187.

Mella J, Biffin A, Radcliffe AG, Stamatakis JD, Steele RJC (1997) Population based audit of colorectal cancer management in two UK health regions. British Journal of Surgery 84: 1731-1736.

Morrin MM, Farrell RJ, Raptopoulos V (2000) Role of virtual computed tomography colonography in patients with colorectal cancers and obstructing colorectal lesions. Diseases of the Colon and Rectum 43: 303-311.

Neugut AI, Garbowski GC, Waye JD et al. (1993) Diagnostic yield of colorectal neoplasia with the use of abdominal pain, change in bowel habits and rectal bleeding. American Journal of Gastroenterology 88: 1179-1184.

Nicholls RJ, Glass R (1985) Coloproctology - Diagnosis and outpatient management. Berlin: Springer-Verlag.

Nicholls RJ, York Mason A, Morson BC, Dixon AK, Fry KI (1982) The clinical staging of rectal cancer. British Journal of Surgery 69: 404-409.

Pescatori M, Maria G, Beltrani B, Mattana M (1982) Site, emergency and duration of symptoms in the prognosis of bowel cancer. Diseases of the Colon and Rectum 25: 33-40.

Quirke P, Durdey P, Dixon MF, Williams NS (1986) The prediction of local recurrence of rectal adenocarcinoma due to inadequate surgical resection. Histopathological study of lateral tumour spread and surgical excision. The Lancet ii: 996-999.

Reeders JAWJ, Bakker AJ, Rosenbusch G (1995) Contemporary radiological examination of the lower gastrointestinal tract. Baillière's Clinical Gastroenterology 9: 701-728.

Rex DK, Lewis BS (1996) Flexible Sigmoidoscopy. Boston, Mass: Blackwell Science.

Rex DK, Rahmani EY, Haseman JH, Lemmel GT, Kaster S, Buckley JS (1997) Relative sensitivity of colonoscopy and barium enema for detection of colorectal cancer in clinical practice. Gastroenterology 112: 17-23.

Rifkin MD, Wechsler RJ (1986) A comparison of computed tomography and endorectal ultrasound in staging rectal cancer. International Journal of Colorectal Disease 1: 219-223.

Rodney W, Dabov G, Orientale E, Reeves W (1993) Sedation associated with a more complex colonoscopy. Journal of Family Practice 36: 394-400.

Royal College of Surgeons of England (1996) Guidelines for the Management of Colorectal Cancer. London: RCSE.

Sands LR, Daniel N (1999) Investigation and examination of a patient with colorectal problems. In: Porrett T, Daniel N (eds), Essential Coloproctology for Nurses. London: Whurr Publishers, pp. 52-75.

Saunders BP, Bell GD, Williams CB, Bladen JS (1995) First clinical results with a real time, electronic imager: an aid to colonoscopy. Gut 36: 913–917.

Schofield PF, Haboubi NY, Martin DF (1993) Highlights in Coloproctology. London: Springer-Verlag.

Schreve RH, Terpstra OT, Ausema L, Lameris JS, van Seiien AJ, Jeekel J (1984) Detection of liver metastases. A prospective study comparing liver enzymes, scintigraphy, ultrasonography and computed tomography. British Journal of Surgery 71: 947–949.

Sonnenberg A, Koch TR (1989) Epidemiology of constipation in the United States. Diseases of the Colon and Rectum 32: 1–8.

Thompson JA, Pond CL, Ellis BG, Beach A, Thompson MR (2000) Rectal bleeding in general and hospital practice: 'the tip of the iceberg'. Colorectal Disease 2: 288–293.

Turnbull RB, Kyle K, Watson FR, Spratt J (1967) Cancer of the colon: the influence of the no touch isolation technique on survival rates. Annals of Surgery 166: 420–427.

UICC (1992) Hermanek P, Sobin LH (eds) TNM Classification of Malignant Tumours, 4th edn, 2nd rev. Berlin: Springer.

UICC Committee on TNM Classification (1966) Malignant Tumours of the Oesophagus, Stomach, Colon and Rectum. Geneva: UICC.

Vining DJ, Gelfand DW, Bechtold RE (1994) Technical feasibility of colon imaging with helical CT and virtual reality [abstract]. AJR American Journal of Roentgenology 162(suppl): 104.

Waizer A, Powsner E, Russo I et al. (1991) Prospective comparative study of magnetic resonance imaging versus transrectal ultrasound for preoperative staging and follow-up of rectal cancer: preliminary report. Diseases of the Colon and Rectum 34: 1068–1072.

Waye JD, Lewis BS, Yessayan S. (1992) Colonoscopy: a prospective report of complications. Journal of Clinical Gastroenterology 15: 347–351.

Whiteford MH, Whiteford HM, Yee LF et al. (2000) Usefulness of FDG-PET scan in the assessment of suspected metastatic or recurrent adenocarcinoma of the colon and rectum. Diseases of the Colon and Rectum 43: 759–767.

Winawer SJ, Fletcher RH, Miller L et al. (1997) Colorectal cancer screening: clinical guidelines and rationale. Gastroenterology 112: 594–642.

Winawer SJ (2000) A comparison of colonoscopy and double contrast barium enema for surveillance after polypectomy. New England Journal of Medicine 342: 1766–1772.

Young GP, St John JB (1991) Selecting an occult blood test for use as a screening tool for large bowel cancer. Frontiers of Gastrointestinal Research 18: 135–156.

Zbar AP, Kmiot WA (1998) Anorectal investigation. In: Phillips RKS (ed.), Colorectal Surgery. London: WB Saunders Co., pp. 1–32.

Chapter 5

Treatments

Shelley Biddles

When the overall survival rate for colorectal cancer is merely 40 per cent, for a potentially curable disease it is essential that any treatments offer optimum prognosis. Surgery is the mainstay treatment for colorectal cancer and therefore should be at the forefront for improving outcomes, using nationally agreed guidelines based on valid research.

In this chapter surgical options are discussed, ranging from the radical and mutilating procedures to the minimally invasive for curative resections to palliation and hepatic surgery. Treatments for colon and rectal malignancies will be considered separately because colon cancer regimens are generally surgical procedures based on tumour location, whereas rectal cancer issues are multifactorial and require greater considerations to ensure best practice. Radiotherapy and chemotherapy in the past decade have been seen to play a more valuable role, especially in rectal cancers, whether as an adjuvant therapy or as palliation. Preoperative oncology treatments are touched on with regard to the rationale for first-line non-surgical treatments and how these impact on surgery.

Recent guidelines by the Association of Coloproctology for Great Britain and Ireland (ACPGB&I, 2001) have made numerous recommendations about treatment options and follow-up, and these are highlighted throughout the chapter.

Principles of surgery

A colorectal surgeon should achieve 'curative resection', i.e. histological confirmation of complete excision and no residual tumour for about 40 per cent of cases (ACPGB&I, 2001). New surgical techniques may now be recommended for selective procedures to effect optimum prognosis; however, there are still traditional principles for cancer surgery:

- Wide resection of the cancer-bearing bowel segment
- Widest feasible excision of the lymphatics draining the cancer-bearing bowel segment

- 'No touch' technique
- Minimum of cancer cell contamination and embolization
- Segmental resection of the colon, removing all possible gross disease with adequate margins and adequate lymph node basin excision to remove regional nodal metastases.

Fisher et al. (1955) demonstrated that this last no-touch isolation technique, in which the blood supply is divided where the tumour is being handled, minimized intravascular and local spread of tumour cells. No significant benefit has been proved in a randomized clinical trial (Wiggers et al., 1988) and it is now thought that the results may be attributable to the adequate lymphatic resection.

Colon cancer: surgical procedures

Colon cancer surgery is predominantly concerned with segmental colonic resection, excision of all gross disease with adequate margins and adequate removal of corresponding lymphatic drainage.

Right hemicolectomy (Figure 5.1)

Carcinoma of the caecum or right side of the colon is usually managed by right hemicolectomy. The operation, via a right transverse or midline incision, consists of resection from the terminal ileum, past the hepatic flexure along to the mid-transverse colon, preserving the middle colic vessels with end-to-end or stapled side-to-side anastomosis and removal of its regional lymphatic drainage.

In this surgical procedure, as with all other colonic resections, the abdomen is explored to determine respectability and to search for synchronous tumours, distant metastases and associated abdominal disease. The small intestinal mesentery and the transverse mesocolon are divided on a line parallel to the superior mesenteric and middle colic arteries, and most of the greater omentum is removed in the resection specimen. The blood vessels are divided and ligated early in the operation, again to avoid dissemination of tumour cells into the portal circulation or the lymphatics.

When the carcinoma is near the ileocaecal valve a substantial segment of the terminal ileum (10–12 cm) with its mesentery should be removed because of the lymphatics along the ileocolic vessels. When the lesion is in the hepatic flexure or mid-transverse colon, less ileum is removed, although careful dissection of the mesentery to the root of the mid-colic from the superior mesenteric is necessary.

Figure 5.1 Right hemicolectomy

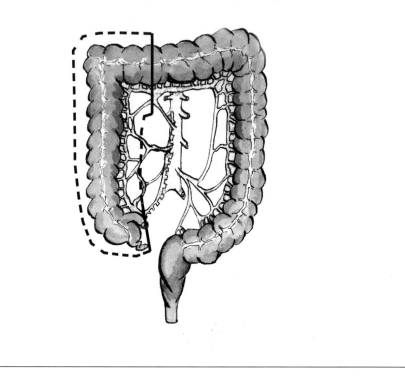

A primary tumour on the right side of the colon is usually resected even if distant metastases have occurred, because prevention of obstruction or anaemia may offer best palliation.

If a patient has an unresectable carcinoma, the obstruction may be bypassed by carrying out a palliative side-to-side anastomosis between the ileum and the transverse colon.

Extended right hemicolectomy (Figure 5.2)

Tumours of the transverse colon and splenic flexure were traditionally managed by segmental resection; however, extended right hemicolectomy is now accepted as a safer option. The procedure is excision of the right colon and a variable length of transverse and descending colon, sacrificing the colic vessels but preserving the inferior mesenteric vessels with ileocolic anastomosis.

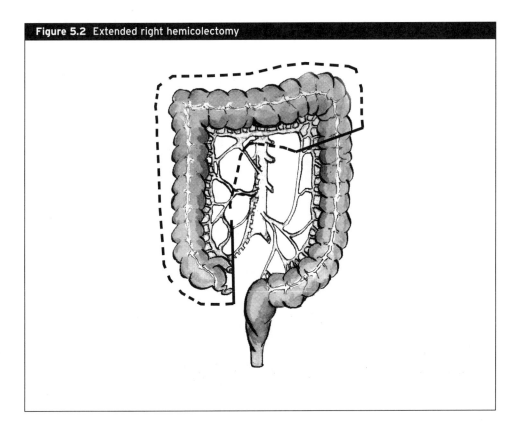

Figure 5.2 Extended right hemicolectomy

Left hemicolectomy (Figure 5.3)

When no intestinal obstruction is present, the treatment of choice for carcinoma of the descending colon is usually managed by left hemicolectomy. Resection, via a midline excision, extends from the middle of the transverse colon to below the sigmoid colon near the origin of the left branch of the middle colic artery. The resection also incorporates excision of a large proportion of the greater omentum and all of the colic mesentery, the left colic artery, the sigmoid vessels and the superior haemorrhoidal artery that supplies the resected bowel. Primary anastomosis is usually performed.

Even when liver metastases are present, this surgery is justified because it gives best palliation. Trephine colostomy formation has little value and has obvious implications regarding body image, quality of life and management/dependency issues.

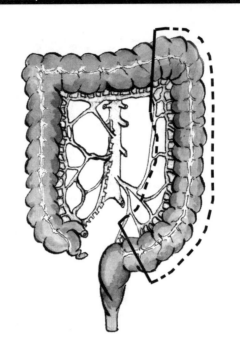

Figure 5.3 Left hemicolectomy

Sigmoid colectomy

Carcinoma of the sigmoid colon is occasionally managed by sigmoid colectomy with primary anastomosis of the descending colon to the rectum, although more frequently anterior resection or left hemicolectomy is the surgical option of choice.

Emergency surgery

Elective surgery is always preferable to help minimize surgical complications and promote optimum prognosis. Eight to nine per cent of patients with colonic cancer present with intestinal obstruction, which equates to approximately 75–80 per cent of all colonic emergencies. Patients with malignant obstruction of the colon are known to have a poorer prognosis stage for stage than those with non-obstructing lesions.

Over the past two decades we have seen a major change in the method of surgical intervention. Previously, when intestinal obstruction was present, the traditional surgical intervention was a three-stage procedure: (1) stoma formation proximal to the obstruction and bowel decompression; (2) resection of the obstructing lesion; and (3) reversal of the stoma.

Nowadays laparotomy with resection tends to be performed with or without a covering stoma where possible, or using a Hartmann's procedure.

Operative mortality and morbidity

Operative morbidity is affected by:

- preoperative health status of the patient
- elective or emergency procedure
- age
- pre-existing health problems of the patient.

Where possible, all colorectal surgery should be performed in the daytime when the full compliment of the colorectal speciality is available. The preoperative anaesthetic assessment is essential, as this directly translates morbidity risk and assists in the preparation for intensive care or high-dependency input.

General early complications of colonic surgery

- Cardiorespiratory:
  - deep vein thrombosis
  - pulmonary embolism
  - chest infection
- Anastomotic leakage
  - more prevalent in left-sided resections
- Sepsis and wound infection
- Urinary retention and infection
- Impotence
- Accidental damage to other organs, e.g. ureters
- Intra-abdominal abscess.

Operative mortality and morbidity are greatly increased with emergency surgery, and when perforation occurs this increases the possibility of:

- wound infections (caused by possible faecal contamination)
- dehiscence

- intraperitoneal abscess
- anastomotic leak
- generalized peritonitis
- systemic sepsis and multiorgan failure.

Late complications

- Anastomotic stricture
- Small bowel or colonic obstruction caused by adhesions
- Tumour recurrence.

The Association of Coloproctology indicates an acceptable mortality rate of between 3 and 7 per cent for elective surgery and between 1 and 25 per cent for emergency procedures. Wound infections should be less than 10 per cent, and anastomotic leak rate should be less than 4 per cent (ACPGB&I, 2001).

Palliation in colonic cancer

If it is technically possible to remove the primary tumour with only a reasonable risk, it is preferable to death from pain, bleeding and faecal discharge of an uncontrolled primary. Obliviously wide clearance of lymphatic drainage is not necessary.

Bypass surgery is indicated when it is not possible or advisable to excise the tumour and the colonic flow is altered, i.e. ileotransverse bypass for unresectable caecal tumour.

At times stoma formation may be indicated to bypass an obstruction but this should be considered only if all other options are not advisable. Trephine or laproscopic stoma formation would be performed to minimize the morbidity risk to the patient and reduce hospitalization.

Stenting

In selected patients with obstructed left colon cancer, non-surgical treatment may be preferred. Deflation of the obstructed colon (often caused by a rectosigmoid lesion) may be achieved by the introduction of a colonic stent to the affected site, using a flexible sigmoidoscope (Keen and Orsay, 1992; Saida et al., 1996).

This should ideally be performed as a joint procedure by the radiologist and colorectal endoscopist. In the patient with a non-resectable tumour and poor prognosis and health status, it improves symptoms without the need (and therefore increased morbidity) for general anaesthesia and probable stoma surgery. For those with acute obstructive symptoms requiring first-line non-surgical treatment, stent insertion may allow temporary relief until surgical excision is appropriate.

Rectal cancer: surgical procedures

Anterior resection (Figure 5.4)

The 1940s and 1950s saw the development of the anterior resection procedure – excision of at least part of the rectum and the sigmoid colon with colorectal anastomosis.

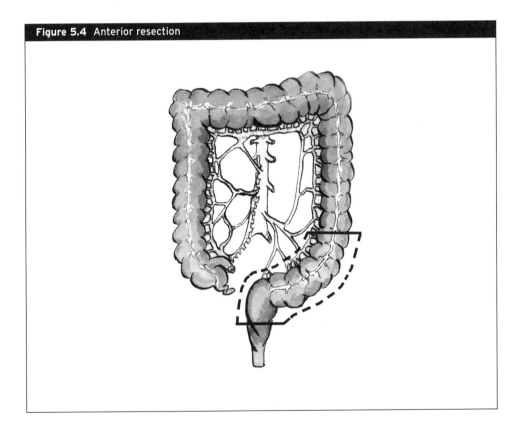

Figure 5.4 Anterior resection

Baker advocated an end-to-side anastomosis as a result of the anatomical physiology. However, the surgery was initially thought to be very controversial and unpopular in colorectal cancer because it was thought to affect local recurrence rates adversely.

Dixon, at the Mayo Clinic, Cleveland, addressed the issue of optimum tumour clearance margins and it was Cuthbert Dukes, in the 1950s, who finally advocated that a 5 cm distal clearance measurement was essential. Current recommendations for tumour clearance measurement are between 1 and 3 cm, although there is no evidence that a distal measurement of 1 cm adversely affects survival, and most will regard this as an acceptable margin for curative resection (Quirke et al., 1986).

Therefore with the advent of new technology, especially the development of stapling guns, and the acceptance of relatively minimal clearance margins, restorative anterior resection is now possible, even in the low-lying rectal tumours.

However, this has brought into question quality of life in relation to functional issues. Anorectal function can be significantly impaired in low anterior resection, with possible autonomic nerve dysfunction. This is commonly known as anterior resection syndrome:

- Increased frequency of defecation
- Urgency and sensitivity regarding the need to defecate
- Fragmentation of stool
- Inability to distinguish flatus from faeces affecting incontinence and soiling.

Another complication is that of anastomotic strictures, which augments the above syndrome and often warrants dilatation via either radiological or surgical procedures.

In 1986, Lazarthes and Parc attempted to address the issue of functional difficulties with the development of colonic reservoir for low anterior resection. The debate continues about whether a colonic pouch offers any benefit to functional competency, although the ACPGB&I (2001) states that this should be considered in low anastomosis. Also, the addition of radiotherapy treatments may augment defecation disturbance and increase sexual dysfunction.

Perioperative anastomotic leakage should be less than 8 per cent (ACPGB&I, 2001) and therefore it is prudent for the surgeon to consider formation of a defunctioning stoma when performing ultra-low anastomosis.

Total mesorectal excision (Figure 5.5)

Traditionally, anterior resection and abdominoperineal excision of the rectum (APER) have produced disappointing results with regard to local recurrence and overall survival for rectal cancer. It may be argued that the use of adjuvant therapies of radiotherapy and chemotherapy has been promoted in an effort to improve these outcomes. Heald questioned the value of traditional rectal surgery and, considering the area of spread in rectal cancer, found that this was usually limited to a field that is encompassed by the integral visceral mesentery of the hindgut, i.e. the mesorectum. When disease is not widely disseminated, resection including the mesorectum offers removal of virtually every tumour satellite and minimizes local recurrence. This procedure described by Heald is now known as total mesorectal excision (TME). Excision of the mesorectum, 'the perfect tumour package' as described by Heald, is where the surgical resection technique, under direct vision, recreates the tissue planes around the intact tumour specimen, preventing tearing and compromising of the clearance margins.

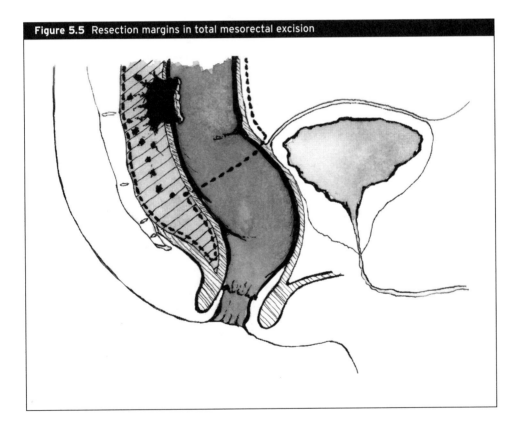

Figure 5.5 Resection margins in total mesorectal excision

Heald et al. (1997) published a study that addressed the efficacy of an extreme policy of sphincter conservation by combining precise TME with low stapling techniques and endoluminal lavage to guard against implantations. It concluded that from a cancer perspective TME offered an improved outcome, suggesting that TME and a temporary defunctioning stoma could treat three-quarters of patients with lower-third rectal cancer. The study also posed the question of whether the wound of abdominoperineal excision might be a prerequisite for perineal recurrence, which may often be caused by implantation. However, functional incompetence versus stoma issues must be carefully addressed when considering ultra-low anterior resection versus abdominoperineal excision of the rectum.

The ACPGB&I (2001) now recommend TME as the surgical procedure for resections within the lower two-thirds of the rectum.

Abdominoperineal excision of rectum (Table 5.6)

This is excision of the whole rectum and anal canal via abdominal and perineal approaches, with the formation of a permanent end-colostomy.

Figure 5.6 Abdominoperineal excision of the rectum

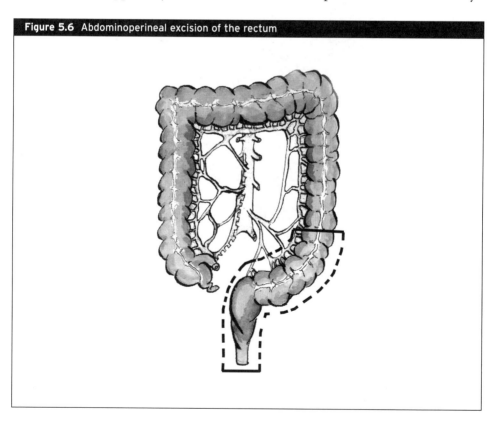

At the turn of the twentieth century, surgery performed for rectal cancer affected a high mortality with almost certain future recurrence. Herbert Allingham (died 1895) was the pioneer of the apple core excision, although he did also perform a colostomy.

Between 1910 and 1920 two surgeons changed the face of colorectal surgery, improving the prognosis of cancer patients. Ernest Miles described his new surgical procedure, which was the foundation for abdominoperineal excision of rectum as we know it. Lockhart Mummery was Miles' contemporary at the time and he described surgery similar to a procedure known as transanal resection of tumour (TART). Miles developed his radical surgery of removing the rectum and the pelvic mesocolon, comprising 'the zone upward spread' in a combined abdominal and perineal approach. The two surgeons, with their varying views, finally agree that the Miles' procedure greatly improved the prognosis of rectal cancer patients and, in 1923, Miles demonstrated that his procedure resulted in an improvement in local recurrence to 29.5 per cent. Miles' abdominoperineal excision of the rectum (APER) then became the gold standard in treatment for rectal cancers up to 15 cm from the anal verge and has certainly been the standard form of surgery for lower-third rectal tumours for over 50 years.

The surgery may continue to be the standard for low rectal tumours but at what cost?

Complications

- Wound dehiscence, in particular perineal dehiscence, especially after preoperative radiotherapy.
- Urinary dysfunctions such as retention, hesitancy and dysuria are common in the short term, particularly in elderly men; however, permanent paresis has been reported in up to 59 per cent after APER (Gerstenberg et al., 1980).
- Sexual dysfunction such as impotence and abnormal ejaculation in men and dyspareunia, decreased vaginal lubrication and lack of orgasm in women. Again, the addition of radiotherapy treatments appears to augment this with a reported effect in about 45 per cent after APER a decade ago, and now a suggested risk factor of 30-70 per cent.
- Stoma problems are uncommon; nevertheless, necrosis, dehiscence and retraction may occur in the perioperative period, with stenosis being a late complication. However, the immense psychosocial impact of mutilating surgery, not withstanding the practical difficulties and implications for some when physical ability may be grossly impaired, cannot be overstated.

There have been wide variations in those performing APER against anterior resection and the Association of Coloproctology recommend that, depending on disease stage at presentation, and if distal clearance of 1 cm can be achieved, anterior resection should be performed; if there is doubt, a further expert opinion should be sought.

Also, the procedure of APER should account for less than 40 per cent of a colorectal surgeon's workload performed for rectal cancers (ACPGB&I, 2001).

Hartmann's procedure (Figure 5.7)

Henri Hartmann described an operation in 1923, which is now defined as a resection of the sigmoid colon, possibly including a length of rectum being excised, with formation of a terminal colostomy and closure of the rectal stump.

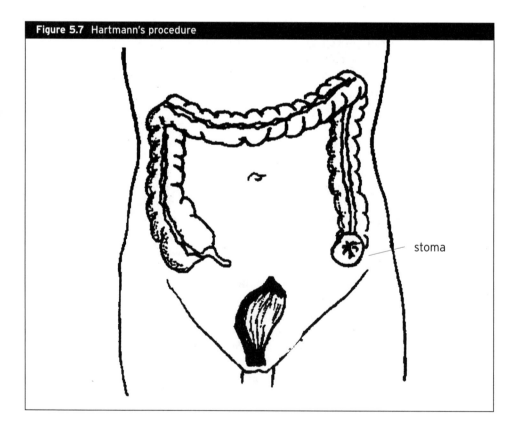

Figure 5.7 Hartmann's procedure

stoma

Traditionally this procedure was indicated for carcinoma of the upper and mid-rectum but this has now largely been superseded by anterior resection. A Hartmann's procedure is generally now performed in the emergency setting, when a patient presents with colonic obstruction or perforation secondary to a carcinoma. Primary anastomosis is often not advisable in these situations. A laparotomy is performed to explore the peritoneal cavity and to identify the primary lesion and any associated disease. The proximal dissection is usually at the last part of the descending colon or sigmoid colon. The diseased segment is, where possible, resected by dividing the distal end with suturing of the remaining rectal stump.

A left iliac colostomy is constructed through a separate incision, which preferably has been predetermined by the colorectal or stoma care nurse specialist in conjunction with the patient, and is clearly marked on the patient's skin.

If the disease is advanced, complete resection with suturing of the rectal stump may not be possible and the tumour may be left *in situ*, draining through the distal rectum. This form of palliative surgery is not recommended because it results in an immeasurably poor quality of life for patients as a result of the physical disruption caused by per rectum tumour drainage.

Complications

- Rectal stump leakage can occur in approximately 10 per cent of cases.
- Stoma complications are uncommon but necrosis may occur perioperatively.
- Wound sepsis, anastomotic leakage and urinary problems are the main complications.
- Anastomotic stenosis can be a late complication.

Sepsis and wound disruption are the more probable complications after emergency surgery and perforation, which in turn may cause small bowel obstruction in rare cases.

Where possible, further surgery for restoration of bowel continuity should be considered. A laparotomy for reversal of Hartmann's procedure will not be without a morbidity/mortality risk and a possible low anastomosis, with the potential of increase in functional disturbances, must be balanced against psychological and autonomy issues. Hartmann's procedure may be considered most prudent in a particular scenario; however, formation of a colostomy, which affects the psychological trauma and practicality of maintenance of independence in a frail and/or palliative patient, must not be underestimated.

Local excision

Transanal local excision does play a significant part in the management of rectal carcinoma, albeit a limited one.

The possibility of cure of selected rectal cancers with minimal morbidity, negligible mortality, and maintenance of normal gastrointestinal and genitourinary function has caused a lot of controversy over the past two decades. Does local excision with curative intent and its current techniques compromise the potential for cure, even for a highly selected group? Selection is critical because the tumour must be anatomically accessible and technically amenable to complete excision with free margins, and have pathology of good or moderate differentiation and be < 3 cm in diameter. If poorly differentiated, lymphatic or vascular invasion is present, or histopathology confirms mucinous or signet ring tumours, local excision will be inadequate and more invasive surgery will be warranted.

The advent of endorectal ultrasonography offers improved accuracy in predicting tumour staging with regard to depth of mural invasion and lymph node involvement. Unfortunately, research indicates that, even with improved scanning techniques, it is still not possible to predict with absolute precision and local excision; certainly, when T2 tumours were treated by this technique, it often resulted in higher than acceptable local recurrence. Salvage surgery is possible, but overall survival is unknown compared with traditional surgical intervention. Tumours involving the muscle coat of the bowel wall have 10–20 per cent of involved nodes in the mesorectum and therefore, at present, curative intent local excision of rectal carcinoma in good-risk patients should probably be limited to those few, highly favourable T1 tumours.

Over the past five years, transanal endoscopic microsurgery (TEMS) has become a popular local excision technique, and published data suggest that this is as effective as traditional transanal resection and may offer greater benefit for polyps in the middle third of the rectum (Steele et al., 1996).

Therefore, when radical resection still produces significant morbidity, mortality and functional deficit, this surgical management is useful for its potential for high-risk patients and very frail patients, and for palliation. Transanal resection of tumour (TART) for patients with significant distant metastases, particularly hepatic and/or peritoneal, or with significant co-morbidity, or for those who present with a rectal carcinoma amenable to local methods of control and unwilling to accept the associated morbidity, may well be preferable to the permanent incapacitation or institutionalization caused by a patient's inability to cope with or manage a stoma.

Laparoscopic surgery

Controversy continues regarding this form of colorectal cancer management; in some research, short-term benefits have been indicated whereas others have indicated that the advantages remain unclear. Advantages to elderly people are reduced complication rate and favourable short-term outcome. Port site recurrence appears to be associated with poor laparoscopic technique (Nduka et al., 1994). In younger patients this form of surgical management of colorectal cancer is not advocated, because long-term benefits/complications are, as yet, unknown. This requires formal identification in a large clinical trial and, at present, these are ongoing.

The recommendations by the ACPGB&I (2001) are that this form of surgery must be performed only by an experienced laparoscopic surgeon and that the patient be entered into a national trial.

Rectal cancer: first-line adjuvant treatment

Although surgery remains the mainstay intervention for colorectal cancer, radiotherapy and chemotherapy are now seen as an integral part of the overall treatment package for selective patients, particularly rectal tumours.

The Swedish trial (1987–90) promoted the use of preoperative short-course radiotherapy in rectal cancer, giving evidence of a reduction rate for local recurrence from 27 per cent to 11 per cent and an increase in overall survival rate from 48 per cent to 58 per cent. This research, however, included surgery performed by general surgeons as well as designated coloproctologists, and where surgery did not include TME.

Individuals performing TME surgery without preoperative radiotherapy have demonstrated lower local recurrence rates than those in the Swedish trial, and therefore this posed the question of whether preoperative radiotherapy actually was a benefit in the light of this new accepted surgical procedure. Further trials have been undertaken and preliminary results (Dutch trial) indicate that there is benefit from preoperative radiotherapy in selective rectal cancer, although this is variable depending on the specific location of the tumour within the rectum.

Nowadays as a result of cancer centre preference or via a clinical trial, many patients with mobile rectal tumours may be offered a 5-day course of radiotherapy to 'sterilize' the tumour bed before surgery. Surgery should be performed within 10 days of the start of this first-line treatment. Delay beyond this time is thought to increase surgical complications greatly.

Side effects experienced by patients are generally minimal, but may include tiredness, diarrhoea and occasionally sore skin. Surgical complications include delayed healing to the perineum and increased risk of wound dehiscence in abdominoperineal excision and higher rates of impotency in both abdominoperineal excision and anterior resection (up to 70 per cent). Long-term complications include fibrosis, small bowel obstruction and, possibly, radiological cancer formation.

Up to 30 per cent of patients with rectal cancer will have locally advanced disease at presentation, which is unresectable or borderline as a result of fixation to adjacent structures, e.g. the prostate and/or the bony pelvis. These fixed or tethered tumours are associated with poor prognosis when compared with mobile tumours, and palliative or incomplete resection has a reported median of 10-month survival. Adjuvant therapy in these cases aims to effect tumour shrinkage and this long-course treatment using synchronous chemotherapy and radiation, known as chemoradiotherapy, is believed to improve the efficacy of radiotherapy by impairing the ability of tumour cells to repair DNA damage.

Treatment consists of 25 fractions of radiotherapy over 33 days in a three-field plan and a chemotherapy regimen of folinic acid and 5-fluorouracil (5FU) on days 1–5 and 29–33.

After this first-line treatment there is a delay of 6–12 weeks before surgical resection, to allow toxicity and subsequent side effects to reduce and possible downstaging of the tumour to occur.

Studies have shown that this is a well-tolerated treatment with good overall compliance and acceptable toxicity, bringing about significant downstaging in about a quarter of cases and rendering over two-thirds resectable.

Side effects and surgical complications described are similar to short-course treatment but with greater intensity.

Therapies are constantly being evaluated and in some regions long-course radiotherapy or chemoradiation has become the first-line treatment of choice for appropriate rectal tumours (ACPGB&I, 2003).

The use of postoperative oncological treatments varies according to pathology staging and location of tumour. Pre- and postoperative treatments are discussed in detail in a later chapter.

Synchronous tumours: surgical management

About 25 per cent of all colorectal cancer patients will present with coexisting polyps in the colon and 3–8 per cent will have synchronous tumours. At present, there are no strict guidelines regarding surgical management, and surgery performed varies greatly, dependent on tumour locations, possible consultant preference, multidisciplinary team agreement and patient considerations of age, health status and preference. The debate about surgical management and the subsequent effect on quality-of-life issues will continue for both synchronous tumours and coexisting polyps. Should extensive colonic and rectal excision be performed, even if simply coexisting polyps are present? Or should we minimize surgical procedures regardless of the coexisting histopathology, and survey by usual investigative procedures at standardized regular intervals?

The following are examples of the range of surgery being performed.

Traditional colorectal surgery

An anterior resection may still be the surgery of choice for synchronous tumours of the sigmoid and mid- or upper rectum.

Subtotal colectomy

For possible synchronous tumours of the descending colon, excision of the descending and sigmoid colon with colorectal anastomosis can be used.

Total colectomy

- Colectomy and anastomosis of ileum to rectum
- Total colectomy and ileostomy and creation of rectal fistula
- Total colectomy and ileostomy with rectal stump.

All are examples of surgery for caecal and sigmoid synchronous tumours.

Panproctocolectomy

- Total excision of the colon with formation of a permanent end-ileostomy
- Possible very low rectal tumour with synchronous tumours elsewhere in the colon.

Stoma formation

Traditionally an end stoma is created in association with Hartmann's procedure or APER, whereas loop stoma formation is performed for diversion or palliation. At present, loop ileostomy tends to be the procedure of choice for diversion and it is estimated that about 20–30 per cent of anterior resections performed will involve formation of a temporary loop ileostomy. This may be the result of anastomotic difficulties at operation or the surgeon's preference for routine protection of the anastomotic site (although the ACPGB&I recommend judicious use of stoma diversion in this instance). Many surgeons will take the following into consideration:

- Low anastomosis is technically more difficult, with greater risk of anastomotic leak.
- Obstructing lesion with inadequate bowel cleansing causes an increased risk of sepsis, leakage, etc.
- Poor colonic vascularity increases anastomotic leak potential.
- When hysterectomy is also performed, closure of the vaginal stump at the same level as the bowel anastomosis increases the risk of rectovaginal fistula.

Stoma formation, whether temporary or permanent, has an immense impact on a patient's rehabilitation. It is also important to note that there are an appreciable number of supposed temporary stomas where reversal is not performed. Quality of life can deteriorate quite markedly and at times this may lead to incapacitation because of the patient's inability to manage the stoma, and even to institutionalization.

Trephine stoma

A trephine procedure was developed for those patients who were not fit enough or did not warrant or want an open procedure. A small incision is made on the abdomen at the elected site (depending on ileostomy or colostomy formation) and the bowel is delivered through the skin wall. The bowel is then either divided using a TA55 stapler, closing the distal end, and the proximal end brought to the surface of the skin to form an end stoma, or a loop stoma is created.

Particularly in the care of colorectal cancer, there are indications for when this procedure is most prudent. In the case of an obstructing fixed rectal cancer where distant metastases have been excluded, it may be necessary to perform a temporary stoma to divert and prevent perforation during long-course chemoradiation therapy, primary resection being performed about six weeks later. Reversal of the stoma may be performed at this operation or deferred to a third-stage surgical procedure. Some patients will occasionally make the choice to decline major surgery, and trephine stoma formation may be an acceptable palliative solution for these patients if the tumour is not amenable to local excision. Naturally, counselling would be offered to ensure full understanding of the implications of their actions, i.e. refusing possible curative resection. In palliation where there is secondary disease and where the lesion is not amenable to localized surgery or where the patient presents a high anaesthetic risk, trephine stoma formation is a viable option.

As major surgery has been avoided, the patient should require less analgesia and normal dietary function will resume much sooner because 'ileus' is less likely to occur, effecting a quicker and safer recovery. Hospital stay may be delayed only as a result of stoma education. Trephine stoma formation is successful in about 90 per cent of appropriate cases with minimal complications. Cicatrization resulting from mucocutaneous dehiscence or stoma stenosis and requiring stoma revision is the most common complication.

The treatment of colorectal hepatic metastases: liver resection

Approximately one-third of colorectal cancer patients in the UK will, at initial presentation, have liver metastases, and each year over 50 per cent of others diagnosed will develop secondary disease in the liver. The mean survival of patients with hepatic metastases without liver surgery is about one year.

Liver resection in appropriate cases is recognized to yield a survival rate of about 30 per cent at 5 years and the past two decades have seen a significant change in attitudes towards patients with hepatic metastases from colorectal cancer because of the results achieved after operative intervention. However, overall the evidence indicates that liver metastases are an indicator for palliation in most cases because liver resection is currently the only curative procedure that can be performed, and this is limited to about 20 per cent of the patients presenting with hepatic secondary disease. Criteria for resection are fairly strict. Evidence of extrahepatic disease is a definite contraindication, as is bilobar disease, significant cardiopulmonary compromise and cirrhosis. Also, often few patients are suitable for this intervention as a result of being unfit for major surgery, or their age or unwillingness to accept the associated morbidity. Liver reserve is rarely a problem because up to 70 per cent can be resected without compromising liver function, although this figure is reduced drastically in the presence of cirrhosis. All possible hepatic metastases should be identified before and confirmed at surgery by intraoperative ultrasonography and resected. Subtotal excision or 'debulking' of the disease is not considered helpful, because it has not been associated with prolongation of life.

Criteria for patient selection and surgical integrity may be quite rigid; this should be endorsed because evidence is now accumulating that within the 5-year survival data indicators of good and bad prognosis may be found. Patients with a single metastasis generally have the best prognosis, with recently published results of 5-year survival rate as high as 60 per cent.

As previously stated patients presenting with disease in both lobes of the liver (bilobar) are generally not suitable candidates for resection. The rationale for this is that the volume of normal liver preserved after resection would not be compatible with life. This has led to the development of a new technique, thermal ablation, which seeks to cause *in situ* destruction of the tumours either intraoperatively (i.e. at primary colorectal surgery) or percutaneously using image guidance.

Most ablative techniques require the placement of a probe into the target tumour, from which energy is released to cause cancer cell death. The following techniques are attractive to the clinician because they destroy metastases, leaving far more normal liver parenchyma than standard resection, and allowing the clinician to treat multiple, bilobar tumours:

- Electrolysis uses the chemicals produced when an electric current is placed between two electrodes. The advantage of this system is that it has as yet caused no bile or blood vessel damage in the ablated volume.
- Microwave ablation uses heat as the cytotoxic medium and can produce very large volumes of ablation more rapidly than any other available ablative technique.
- High-powered focused ultrasonography.
- Cryotherapy.
- Radiofrequency ablation.
- Interstitial laser photocoagulation.

These techniques have promising short-term results when used to treat patients with unresectable liver tumours. However, as yet there is no evidence to support the contention that these new techniques influence overall survival in colorectal cancer patients; consequently clinical randomized controlled trials need to be undertaken to audit the effectiveness of these treatments.

The development and collaboration of colorectal and hepatobiliary multidisciplinary teams now allow more patients to be assessed for liver surgery, promoting new operative techniques and extending the boundaries for potential cure.

Anal cancer

Anal carcinoma is still relatively rare in Western society; Northover (1993) states that there are 100 cases of colorectal cancer for each new anal tumour. Most cases are of epidermoid origin, with 80 per cent being squamous cell carcinoma.

Anal tumours can be categorized into those in the anal canal, at or above the dentate line, or those at the anal margin, below the dentate line. Invasion into the anal sphincters may occur, with spread to the superior haemorrhoidal lymph nodes in the case of a tumour above the dentate line, or to the inguinal lymph nodes for those tumours below the dentate line.

Anal tumours manifest as ulcers or proliferate growths with ulceration present; as they advance they become hard and fixed. Histologically they vary from being well-differentiated, keratinizing, large-cell tumours to poorly differentiated, non-keratinizing, small-cell tumours in the upper anal canal. One major difference between anal and colorectal cancer is that anal tumours spread mainly only within the pelvis and rarely have distant spread.

Traditionally, treatment of anal cancer has been surgical intervention by radical APER. However, in the 1970s an American report suggested chemotherapy treatment as a possible cure. At the same time, Papillon in France reported on the benefits of radiotherapy with early rectal tumours and, following this, others suggested similar benefits to anal tumours. Now radiation therapy, or combined chemoradiation in particular, has become the more optimal treatment of choice. A British study in 1988 (Geh, 1988) reported where combination radiation and chemotherapy resulted in a response rate of 80–90 per cent and a 5-year survival rate of about 83 per cent. This combination therapy of about six weeks is arduous for the patient but is now considered the most appropriate first-line treatment. Therefore, most patients undergoing chemoradiation should not require any surgical intervention after biopsy confirmation. A temporary trephine loop stoma may be necessary in isolated cases, if the risk of obstruction is high before the start of treatment or if skin excoriation occurs during treatment, which becomes unmanageable. If the tumour was initially treated by local excision, chemoradiation should be considered before radical surgery.

Surgical intervention of abdominoperineal excision should be reserved for residual or recurrent disease, permanent anal sphincter damage or the complications of chemoradiation therapy.

Follow-up

Surveillance or 'follow-up' of patients undergoing curative resection for primary colorectal cancer is controversial. Sugarbaker et al. (1998) determined from a prospective trial that most colorectal cancer recurrence occurs within two years of the primary resection. Of patients, 85 per cent had a recurrence within 30 months, with a median time of 17 months, and all sites recurrence developed at the same time.

Among the key aims of surveillance are the early detection of recurrent disease or metachronous tumours, amenable to cure, and the provision of psychological support and audit. Traditionally all patients receive 'follow-up' from a surgical and/or oncology team and, despite the lack of clear evidence, this tends to be non-discriminate of disease staging and diverse in its pathway of surveillance management from clinician to clinician, hospital to hospital.

The 'practice' of follow-up for colorectal cancer is immensely diverse throughout the UK, in both timings and investigative procedures. Enthusiasts of intensive medical follow-up believe that this route assists early detection of recurrence, encouraging early intervention, and is a proactive pathway of care aiming for reduction in mortality. Others, however, will argue that this, as yet, remains unproven.

Many investigative procedures now exist, but again there is no consensus about their value. Hospitals, too, have an inconsistency regarding available investigative resources and the demands on these facilities. Therefore, is it not understandable that many clinicians have tended to devise their own protocols?

The New NHS Cancer Plan (DoH, 2000) encourages the advancement of personal choice and direct booking. As life becomes more hectic, is it acceptable to expect patients to take time out to visit an outpatients clinic where the waiting time is invariably longer than that of the medical consultation? Outpatient appointments are an integral part of the patient's pathway of care and many acknowledge the important aspect of that care; however, as previously demonstrated, there is little evidence to support that it is of physical/survival benefit, although some studies have indicated psychological benefits.

The Government and the ACPGB&I guidelines recommend the following investigations:

- Colonoscopy to detect metachronous or recurrent tumours in asymptomatic patients. As yet there is no evidence that this investigation improves survival; it is, however, acknowledged that it detects a high yield of treatable adenomatous polyps and cancer.

- Regular hepatic imaging by ultrasonography or computed tomography may detect operable liver metastases.

Controversy remains about the concentration of the blood tumour marker carcinoembryonic antigen. Some, often oncologists, regard this as a useful tool to prompt intensive investigation when the marker is raised. Others will argue that often this simply causes anxiety to the patient because recurrence often cannot be found at that time or, if found, salvage surgery may not be possible.

At present the detection rate of recurrent disease with possible salvage surgery probably has less than a 2 per cent success rate. Therefore, the major disadvantage of follow-up is the ability to demonstrate that this is associated with a significant improvement in overall survival rate.

References

Association of Coloproctology of Great Britain and Ireland (2001) Guidelines for the Management of Colorectal Cancer. London: ACPGB&I.

Boulos PB, Wexner SD (2000) Colorectal Surgery. Philadelphia: WB Saunders.

Burkitt HG, Quick CRG, Gatt D (1996) Essential Surgery. Edinburgh: Churchill Livingstone.

Cushieri A, Hennessy TPJ, Greenhalgh RA, Rowley DI, Grace PA (1996) Clinical Surgery. Oxford: Blackwell Science.

Deans GT, Spence RAJ, Love AHG (1998) Colorectal Disease for Physicians and Surgeons. Oxford: Oxford University Press.

Department of Health (2000) The NHS National Cancer Plan. London: HMSO.

Forest APM, Carter DC, Macleod IB (1995) Principles and Practice of Surgery. Edinburgh: Churchill Livingstone.

Goligher J (1984) Surgery of the Anus, Rectum, and Colon. London: Baillière Tindall.

Heald RJ (1988) The 'holy plane' of rectal surgery. Journal of the Royal Society of Medicine 81: 503-508.

Heald RJ, Husband EM, Ryall RDH (1982) The mesorectum in rectal cancer surgery – the clue to pelvic recurrence? British Journal of Surgery 69: 613-616.

Hobsley M (1986) Pathways in Surgical Management. London: Arnold,

Jones PF, Siwek RJP (1986) Colorectal Surgery. Wolfe Medical Publications Ltd.

Lipkin M., Good RA (1978) Gastrointestinal Tract Cancer. New York: Plenum Publishing Corporation.

McArdle C (2000) Effectiveness of follow up. British Medical Journal 321: 1332-1335.

McCulloch P, Kingsnorth A (1996) Management of Gastrointestinal Cancer. London: BMJ Publishing Group.

Misiewicz JJ, Bartram CI, Cotton RB, Mee AS, Price AB, Thompson RPH (1988) Diseases of the Colon and Rectum. London: Gower Medical Publishing.

Nduka CC, Monson JRT, Menzies-Gow N et al. (1994) Abdominal wall metastases following laparoscopy. British Journal of Surgery 81: 648-652.

Porrett,T, Daniel N (1999) Essential Coloproctology for Nurses. London: Whurr Publishers.

Quirke P, Durdey P, Dixon MF et al. (1986) Local recurrence of rectal adenocarcinoma due to inadequate surgical resection: histopathological study of lateral tumour spread and surgical excision. The Lancet ii: 996-999.

Rob & Smith (1993) Operative Surgery. Surgery of the colon rectum and anus. Oxford: Butterworth-Heinemann.

Rosin D (1994) Minimal Access General Surgery. Oxford: Radcliffe Medical Press Ltd.

Schoemaker D, Touli J, Black R, Giles L (1998) Yearly colonoscopy, liver CT and chest radiography. Do not influence 5-year survival of colorectal patients. Gastroenterology 114: 7-14.

Steele RJC, Hirshman MJ, Mortensen NJMcC et al. (1996) Trans anal endoscopic micro-surgery - initial experience from three centres in the UK. British Journal of Surgery 83: 207-210.

Sugarbaker PH, Gianola FJ, Dwyer A et al. (1987) A simplified plan for follow-up of patients with colon and rectal cancer supported by prospective studies of laboratory and radiological results. Surgery 102: 79-87.

Wiggers T, Arends JW, Volovics A (1988) Regression analysis of prognostic factors in colorectal cancer after curative resections. Diseases of the Colon and Rectum 31: 33-41.

Williams NS (1996) Colorectal Cancer. Edinburgh: Churchill Livingstone.

Chapter 6

Consequences of rectal surgery

Jane Winney

> It is the province of knowledge to speak, and it is the privilege of wisdom to listen.
>
> Holmes

The aim of this chapter is to raise awareness of the physical, psychological and social impact of rectal surgery and the change of bowel function as a result of surgery, and how this may affect an individual's body image and sexual function.

Psychological issues related to cancer and body image are discussed and strategies for assessment and support, and useful interventions, examined. In exploring some of the psychological issues around bowel surgery it must be emphasized that these do not stand alone and are inextricably interwoven with physical, social, spiritual and sexual health. Therefore, a holistic approach to care is the key to providing emotional support through these traumatic life experiences. These topics are viewed against the backdrop of the political agenda. Throughout this chapter the term 'patient' is used to describe those people accessing any of the services of health care professionals in any setting.

Patient choice and informed consent

The political agenda of the day demands that patients must be involved in the decision-making process (Department of Health, 1996, 1999, 2000). However, work by Sanders and Skevinton (2003) concludes that most bowel cancer patients preferred a limited role in the decision-making process and wished to delegate responsibility to the clinician, although they considered that they were active participants within the consultations and accepted the ultimate responsibility of deciding to accept or refuse treatment. After reviewing the results of the Audit Commission (1993) Kinrade (2002) questions whether patients are in a position to give informed consent if they do not have access to written or alternative information to supplement the oral consultation. All involved in caring for people undergoing bowel surgery must have a fundamental understanding of the nature and impact of the proposed operation to ensure informed consent for treatment. This must include the risks as well as the benefits; Dimond (1999) asserts that where there is a duty of care, this includes the duty to inform. Before surgery, preoperative information not only is essential for informed consent but also helps to reduce anxiety levels (Jacoby et al., 1999). Therefore, details of the planned operation and any potential complications must be discussed and treatment options given. *The Patient's Charter* (DoH, 1990) states that patients have the right to clear information about proposed treatments and any risks involved. The importance of this is highlighted in *The NHS Plan* (DoH, 2000), which aims at making information readily available to patients, relatives and carers. The Audit Commission (1993) concluded that there was a lack of provision of patient information for ethnic minorities in a language other than English and too few leaflets available in large print for the partially sighted. In this new millennium and our multicultural society these findings are no longer acceptable and pose a significant challenge to informed consent.

For consent to be valid, the person must be mentally competent and understand the invasion of the intended treatment or procedure (Dimond, 2002). Informed consent is a process (Jacoby et al., 1999; Wallace, 2000; Dimond, 2002) and all who engage in the information-giving are a part of that process and must be confident and competent to explain to the patient the proposed procedure in words that the individual can understand. Any questions relating to care must be answered fully and accurately or referred to the appropriate person (Dimond, 2002). The consent must be given without duress (Wallace, 2000). Gaining consent from patients is an integral part of everyday practice for all health care professionals (McKee, 1999) and is based on principles of autonomy, which decree that people have the right to full disclosure of information including recognized complications in order to make an informed decision and assume responsibility for the consequences of that decision (Walshe and Offen, 2001; Fortes Mayer, 2001). This chapter sets out to help answer some of those questions in connection with rectal surgery.

For those who are unable to represent themselves, the clinician responsible for the case may instigate treatment if it is deemed to be in the patient's best interest; however, lay advocacy should also be considered. Professionals involved in the delivery of care, however well intentioned, cannot be unbiased, because they will inevitably be influenced by a professional, managerial or political agenda. In seeking independent representation, it is worthy of note that legally the next of kin can neither consent nor refuse consent to treatment.

The underlying gastrointestinal pathology may well have an impact on the acceptance of the need for surgery. This reinforces the importance, for all those in contact with the patients as they progress through various departments and stages of investigation and treatment, to understand the nature of the disease, the proposed treatment and any complications that may arise, and to keep the patient appropriately informed (DoH, 2002). During times when the individual is feeling unwell or shocked, he or she will not retain all the oral information given, and supporting written, audio or video tapes are helpful in underpinning the oral consultation.

Body image and sexuality

To appreciate some of the psychological trauma associated with rectal surgery, issues around body image and sexuality need to be examined.

To begin with, it is worth exploring what is defined and accepted as body image and sexuality. According to McKenzie (1988) the expression of body image and sexuality are indivisible in both health and sickness. The following represents a range of opinion from the literature. Body image may be described as the way that we perceive ourselves, and any disruption to this will have a psychological influence on our personal well-being. We are not born with a body image; this is acquired from early childhood as babies begin to develop a sense of individual identity. Pettitt (1980) asserts that this process begins when a baby starts to become mobile and realizes that he or she is a separate entity from the mother, and increases as the senses of touch, hearing and smell develop. From the age of about 2 years, toddlers are urged to evacuate their bowels and urinary systems in private and are taught that to do otherwise is antisocial and unacceptable. Praise and positive reinforcement are encouraged when they gain control over their anal and bladder sphincters. Body image is inextricably linked to these early developmental years and subsequent environmental factors and social influences and attitudes. Thus, the devastation experienced with the loss of control of what can be viewed as a basic bodily function cannot be overestimated. This is particularly relevant to those who undergo surgery resulting in stoma formation. It is estimated that 20 per cent of this group of patients will suffer symptoms of psychological stress and distress in the postoperative period (White and Unwin, 1998).

Sexuality is difficult to define because, although it is connected, it is not exclusively about sexual function. Sexuality is linked to femininity and masculinity. Vans Oijen and Charnock (1995) caution against having a simplistic or definitive view of sexuality. They challenge the view from the sociological vantage point that claims that sexuality consists of social interaction, social environment, culture and learnt behaviour. However, all these factors play a part in sexuality and, as Burke and Walsh (1992) point out, everyone has sexual feelings, attitudes and beliefs, and yet each individual experiences sexuality through a totally individual perspective, regardless of age or gender. Vans Oijen and Charnock (1995) assert that understanding the concept of sexuality is dependent on a degree of self-awareness and knowledge of different sexual practices. To enable a full assessment of patients' needs, health care professionals must examine their own personal attitudes and beliefs to deliver non-judgemental supportive care. With sensitivity and understanding, all health care workers can help individuals to reconcile the surgically induced loss and make adjustments to adapt to a new situation. Indeed, it should not be seen as one person's responsibility to provide emotional support but more a team culpability (Walsh, 1995). Friends, family and carers will play a part in the adjustment programme, because their attitude and response will affect the acceptability of the new situation, e.g. if a nurse, friend or relative shows distaste at an offensive wound or newly formed stoma this may engender a feeling of rejection, isolation, depression and non-desirability. Many of these responses will be implied by look or body language rather than by verbal reaction, and once made cannot be retracted.

The inevitable scar of any surgical procedure will have a psychological effect, which at times is viewed as evidence of a bodily mutilation. For some this will require adjustment in clothing, particularly men who go shirtless in warm weather or women who usually wear scant swimwear. Others will see that it has a positive sign of renewed life, the price they have paid for health. These views are often expressed by the same person at different times, which highlights the implicit danger of making assumptions about a patient's response, and strengthens the need for individual assessment at each contact. For those who have surgery for a malignant condition, the scar may stand as a constant reminder of the disease and represent a threat to life and the future (Burt, 1995). Knowledge of the specific operation and its effect on bowel function and the exploration of how this impacts on the individual will help in the early identification of psychological morbidity so that appropriate intervention can be made.

Based on real experiences, the impact of rectal surgery is now explored using case studies to illustrate aspects of care.

Scenario 1

Mr Black was a 60-year-old self-employed construction engineer. He had adult children and young grandchildren from a previous marriage and a 12-year-old daughter with his present wife, who was 15 years his junior. He was proud of his physique; he played squash and regularly attended the gym to maintain the muscle tone of his tanned body. He consulted his GP because his normally regular bowel habit had changed to looser, more frequent stools, which was inconveniencing his work routine. He felt well and was confident that all he needed was a prescription for medication to regulate his bowel movement. He was surprised, but not unduly concerned, when his GP referred him for further investigations, and during this phase adopted the view that he did not have any serious condition until it was proven otherwise. He continued to work and pursue his leisure activities as normal. This coping mechanism served him well for this period of time. The result of his investigations revealed a low rectal cancer and this news was broken to him and his wife by the surgeon. His response to this was one of total disbelief; he reasoned that he could not feel so well and have a serious condition that would require such drastic treatment.

Treatment modalities for rectal cancer include surgery, radiotherapy and chemotherapy; frequently a combination of all three is used. Preoperative radiotherapy may be given but surgery is the foundation of treatment and the only prospect of a cure. Removal of the rectum involves an abdominal and perineal incision; it is important that the patient is told this and that he or she will no longer have an anus but will require a permanent colostomy to eliminate body waste. It is acknowledged that the diagnosis of cancer alone has a considerable effect on the psychological health of the patient and carers, adversely affecting quality of life (Fallowfield et al., 2001). This distress may manifest itself in a wide range of emotions. It was important that Mr Black was given the time and the space to express these emotions in a safe environment. Health care professionals need training and support to cope with the outpouring of emotion and distress during these episodes. At such times, the giving of essential information to ensure informed consent may not be heard or assimilated; for that reason, no assumption about the level of understanding can be made and an opportunity for further discussion must be offered.

The wide excision of the tumour takes in the removal of surrounding supporting structures including the lymph nodes that drain this area. As discussed elsewhere, the histological examination and subsequent findings determine future management and so the patient is faced with a cancer diagnosis, major surgery, a permanent stoma and the possibility of postoperative chemotherapy. In addition to this, the operation may result in nerve damage causing sexual and/or urinary dysfunction. Assessment of erectile dysfunction is complex and often requires referral for specialist help and management; however, it is the role of all team members to be aware of the potential difficulties and to be available and open to discussion so that the problem does not go unrecognized and that help is not inadvertently denied (Borwell, 1997). As Taylor (1994) points out, stomas are not a general subject of conversation and may be viewed as 'not nice to talk about' and that, in addition to this, health carers may find themselves floundering with the issue of sexual dysfunction. In her review of the literature Dorey (2002) identifies seven assessment components for erectile dysfunction:

- rigidity
- vascular flow
- nerve conductivity
- intracavernosal pressure
- ischiocavernosus muscle power
- partner satisfaction
- quality of life.

Studies report ongoing misery seriously affecting many aspects of quality of life for those with colorectal cancer (Sprangers et al., 1995), particularly in those who have a stoma. Sprangers et al.'s study suggested that psychological dysfunction relating to low self-esteem, stigma, loneliness and depression, as well as suicidal thoughts, is greater in those with a stoma than in those with intact anal sphincters. However, both groups reported a significant impact on the quality of life from limitations placed on physical, psychological, social and sexual function as a result of treatment.

Mr Black accepted the proposed treatment plan but displayed a range of emotions at various times, and over a period of time expressed his feelings, anxieties and concerns. He felt vulnerable and 'out of control of my own situation'; this was particularly difficult because he saw his role in life as the strong family leader and provider. He had an unfounded and irrational belief that his wife would no longer find him good-looking and may 'look for a younger bloke elsewhere'. As he faced his own mortality he reproached himself for marrying a woman so much younger and convinced himself that he would not live to see his youngest daughter grow up, which was a cause of great distress to him. In his belief that the colostomy would be obvious to everyone and form the focus of attention, he would not contemplate resuming his leisure activities. He viewed the colostomy as antisocial and was sure that, when it functioned in company, there was a malodorous smell apparent to all. These thoughts are not unusual, and the psychological adjustment and social integration challenges faced by those who have stoma surgery is well documented (Devlin and Plant, 1971; Follick, Smith and Turk, 1984; White, 1998). Unable to control the unpredictable function of the stoma left him feeling dirty and unclean. In spite of attempted reassurance, he became depressed and withdrawn. His wife felt bereft and confused as she absorbed much of his frustration and anger and struggled with her own emotions. She found it difficult to cope when he expressed the view that his life, having changed beyond recognition to him, was not worth living. He was unable to work for many months and thus unable to provide for his family; he felt a physical and financial burden to them. His daughter became disruptive at school as she struggled to understand the total disruption to her world.

This example is not unusual and serves to underpin the notion that the physical, psychological and social elements are inextricably intertwined and affect the entire family group, not just the person at the centre of care. Eventually Mr Black chose to manage his colostomy with colostomy irrigation. Irrigation is an option for colostomy management; this works by stimulating peristaltic movement and faecal evacuation by instilling water into the colon. The water is fed into the colon through a length of tubing attached to a water reservoir and a cone; it effectively empties the descending colon and distal third of the transverse colon. The procedure is performed once every 24–48 hours, leaving the patient free of bowel actions between times. This helped psychologically because Mr Black felt that he had regained some control over his bodily function; to him this made it more socially acceptable. With the help of the clinical psychologist he resumed work but maintains that his life has been irrevocably damaged through this experience. This reflects Laurent's (1999) view, who argues that nurses play a vital role in this adjustment process.

The learning point here is for health care professionals to accept that emotional pain is often deep and that a team approach to care is essential to minimize the psychosocial impact and enable the maximization of the health potential, so that the individual can regain an acceptable level of function. As Salter and Ziekenhuis (1998) point out, the pain and outrage at altered body image may continue; they make reference to Lindsey, whose view, endorsed by the author, is that the identity change will become increasingly complicated as patients travel through the illness trajectory, reaffirming the need for sensitive, skilled assessment and support from all involved in their care.

Scenario 2

Mr Green is a 43-year-old unemployed divorcee. His cancer was in the upper third of the rectum, and he accepted the operation of low anterior resection with a temporary ileostomy. He maintained a good sense of humour throughout, even when he suffered from chemotherapy side effects. During this time he appreciated the contact with a wide range of professionals who also helped to fill a social void. His attitude was very pragmatic; he was clear that 'If you tell me what is going on I may not like it, but at least I will be able to understand and cope.' He managed his temporary ileostomy well, showing an early interest in the practical management of stomal toilet, and at all times rationalizing that it was not a permanent situation and that life would improve once the stoma was reversed. Using the temporary status of the stoma as the focus for coping is a concern, as a study by Bailey et al. (2003) suggests that, for a variety of reasons, an estimated 8 per cent of stomas raised with anterior resection will become permanent and that patients should be informed of this risk. Unfortunately, the wide excision of the cancer had left a legacy of nerve damage, which manifested itself as intermittent faecal incontinence, and urological and sexual disturbances. Before his surgery he had formed an illicit relationship with a married friend. Although he was still in contact with the woman, he felt he should not seek to progress the relationship, as he had intended because it 'wouldn't be fair to her to expect her to leave her husband for someone who wouldn't be able to have decent sex'. The pressure to prove his sexual prowess in stolen moments intensified the problem, which was further compounded by erratic faecal incontinence.

Through support and encouragement he was able to articulate these difficulties and with the help of medication he was able to effect an erection to the mutual satisfaction of both him and his partner. He accepted the continence limitations, stating that this for him was preferable to a permanent ileostomy. The learning point that this scenario offers is to highlight the importance of giving people choices to help them accept an option that they feel is acceptable to them, remembering that in many situations there may not be an ideal solution.

Scenario 3

Mrs White is a 26-year-old woman; she had an emergency subtotal colectomy and formation of ileostomy for perforation of her bowel as a result of ulcerative colitis. From the outset she had a practical approach to her stomal management, expressing interest in the various appliances. She had recently married since having the operation. Subsequently, after much discussion, she has decided against the option of surgery to create an internal pouch from small bowel with an anastomosis to the anal canal, which would obviate the need for a permanent ileostomy, and elected to have her rectum removed. Discussions took place around the risks and benefits of both surgical procedures. She met with people who had chosen both options and finally based her decision on the following: she wanted to be as free as possible from hospital follow-up. If she had chosen the pouch option this would require regular follow-up to ensure that no malignant changes were occurring at the site of the anastomosis. She would still evacuate her bowels three to five times per 24 hours and might intermittently be incontinent, particularly of mucus. This is common in the first year after surgery, especially at night. She was principally concerned about the prospect of this seepage of mucus occurring during sexual intercourse. She adopted the view that she felt confident with her stoma and, as she had married since its acquisition, felt secure in the knowledge that her husband still found her physically attractive and desirable. She had returned to work as youth leader and pursued her hobby of horse riding. She viewed the stoma as an occasional nuisance but refused to allow it to dominate her life.

For her, the benefits of surgery to be free of her stoma did not justify the additional operations, follow-up and possibility of anal incontinence, even temporarily. To remove the rectum involves an abdominal and perineal incision. Her main questions were around her future aspirations for parenthood and her ability to have a vaginal delivery. She was assured that this was possible but that it should be closely monitored to enable early intervention if there was undue stress on the perineal scar. After her surgery she experienced a period of dyspareunia and low libido. This is an acknowledged effect of rectal surgery and had been explained to her before the operation. Dyspareunia may be caused by fibrosis of the pelvic floor or posterior wall of the vagina, causing discomfort as the penis connects with rigid scar tissue during penetration. Sometimes an adjustment of position during intercourse can minimize the discomfort. However, the fear of discomfort can result in hesitancy to engage in sexual activity, reluctance to discuss the issue, and consequently tension in the relationship. This tension may also exacerbate the degree of discomfort, reinforcing the negative fear. Awareness of any difficulties by health care professionals will allow timely help for resolution of the difficulties but must be dealt with skilfully and sensitively.

Mrs White also found the tension of the perineal scar painful when she tried to resume her hobby of horse riding; this eased over a period of time with the application of a lanolin-rich cream. Following removal of the rectum, scar tissue along the nerve pathway can create the sensation of a full rectum and an urge to defecate. These 'phantom rectum' feelings can be a source of distress but often diminish over a period of time. During this period she questioned the validity of her choice. There were times when she felt that her femininity had been assaulted and saw the stoma as a phallic symbol, particularly during times of peristaltic movement when the stoma became erect. This was a difficult time for both her and her husband as she rejected his attempts to understand and reassure her.

Conversely, Mr Brown, a 33-year-old office manager whose hobby was sailing, decided to choose the option of pouch surgery. He was a divorcee with a close relationship with his two adolescent children. He was not in a personal relationship at the time of surgery but his ex-wife, who had remarried, was very supportive. He had a temporary ileostomy to reduce the risk of anastomotic leak, which he viewed as the ultimate mutilation of his body. In the ensuing two years after closure of the ileostomy, he suffered from episodes of pouchitis and nocturnal leakage of mucus; in turn this caused some perianal soreness which was exacerbated by the pad that he wore 'just in case of an accident'. He avoided close female relationships and agonized about the fear of sexual failure and rejection. He kept away from community gatherings because he was afraid of anal leakage, which he was convinced would be malodorous. For a period of time he became emotionally withdrawn and socially isolated. Superficially he functioned well at work and, to the casual observer, the obvious improvement in his physical well-being was evidence of a full recovery. This scenario illustrates the need for deeper exploration by health care professionals in order to identify difficulties and provide the necessary support and care. Strategies for this are discussed later.

These scenarios illustrate some of the common themes that emerge when caring for people who have undergone rectal surgery.

Patient assessment

Patient assessment and care planning by the team are crucial and, according to Kelman and Minkler (1985), also cost-effective. The benefit of creating opportunities to allow the expression of feelings and fears cannot be overestimated. The following is an offering of strategies that may be useful. In seeking to help those who have experienced total disruption in all aspects of their daily life through rectal surgery, to make a healthy adaptation to changes in body image it is worth remembering Price (1990), who claims that there are three components to body image:

- Body reality: the way the body actually is, e.g. disfigured by surgery.
- Body ideal: the way in which the person would like to look, e.g. perfectly proportioned without any scars.
- Body presentation: the way in which the person tries to match the body reality and ideal, e.g. through appearance and dress.

Body presentation strives to bring together the elements of body reality and body ideal. In the early post-discharge days, this may mean exploring modifications of clothing to accommodate, for instance, a newly formed stoma. Men may find the wearing of braces more comfortable than a belt; however, if this is not usually a part of the wardrobe, it potentially serves as a constant reminder of the life-changing event. Both men and women may seek to hide abdominal scars that are florid and visible when wearing swimwear. This change process is accompanied by all the natural fears of new situations, and takes time. During this period constant reassurance from family, friends and professionals that they are valued for who they are, and not for what they look like will help, the recovery process. Walsh (1995), cited by Salter and Ziekenhuis (1998), asserts that multiple adjustment demands are placed on those who undergo stoma surgery. Postoperatively the setting of short-term goals is the key to survival; feedback, encouragement and positive reinforcement help to re-establish dented self-esteem. Acknowledgement of small achievements such as washing and dressing themselves is very powerful in starting the programme of re-establishing independence and life fulfilment.

Active listening

Active listening is more than just hearing, demanding a complex mental process, energy and discipline. It is a learned skill. Koshy (1989) asserts that active listening is an essential skill of a wide range of work activities and is especially important for nursing care, and goes on to describe it as 'the process of receiving and assimilating ideas and information from verbal and non-verbal messages and responding appropriately'. According to Hargie and McCartan (1986), of the 70–80 per cent of time spent in verbal activities in the course of a working day, 45 per cent or more of that time is spent listening. The non-verbal cues are often the most valuable when establishing the underlying feelings and response to disfiguring surgery. Koshy (1989) offers the following framework for this:

- The use of silence
- Accepting
- Restating
- Rephrasing
- Clarifying
- Reflecting
- Summarizing
- Awareness of own prejudices
- Giving undivided attention.

The body posture, tone of voice and avoidance of eye contact all give clues to the inner turmoil and distress. Listening to the individual's entire story, while talking as little as possible, can be therapeutic in itself, as well as using open-ended questions to encourage free expression. An encouraging, non-judgemental response with a smile or a nod elicits valuable insight into feelings, perceptions and misconceptions. To rephrase or repeat what has been said is helpful in establishing understanding of what has been verbalized.

Full assessment is incomplete if considerations of cultural and religious beliefs are ignored, because these are key to who we are and how we view the world. In coping with the physical changes in body function and the inevitable psychological impact, the setting of achievable goals helps the gradual adjustment process, which continues long after discharge from hospital. Corner, cited by Salter and Ziekenhuis (1998), suggests that supportive care should be participative, empowering and collaborative, reflecting more of a partnership between health care professionals and patients – an approach that is advocated in *The NHS Plan* (DoH, 2000) and endorsed by the Nursing and Midwifery Council (2002) in the code of professional conduct for nurses. To achieve this demands not only a change in approach and culture from the traditional paternalistic attitude entrenched in the NHS, but also the development of negotiating, communicating and assessment skills by all health care workers. In essence, apart from attending to the physical needs, patients will need to be informed about the physiological changes that will result from the surgical intervention. This advice and support should be constant and consistent along the care pathway, so that understanding can be checked and knowledge reinforced.

Assessment and management of sexual dysfunction will hinge first around identifying the problem or difficulty:

- Lack of libido (both sexes)
- Male:
  - erectile dysfunction
  - ejaculation difficulties (retarded/premature)
- Female:
  - vaginismus
  - dyspareunia
  - anorgasmia.

Second, it deals with those who are within the sphere of the health care professional involved, and refers on those that aren't to a suitably qualified person. Openness, preoperative counselling and encouragement of free expression of feelings will help. Management of erectile dysfunction may include oral medication, injections into the penis to effect an erection, intraurethral pellets, penile implants, vacuum pumps and sex aids. Relationship counselling is a prerequisite to prescribing a course of treatment. Although many of these strategies are effective in producing an erect penis, there is often a loss or change of penile sensation, and some loss of spontaneity in sexual function; therefore, counselling and ongoing support are essential through the adaptation period. In addition to oral medication, oestrogen creams, sex aids and sexual repositioning, the successful management of female sexual dysfunction is also dependent on skilled counselling and support.

Conclusion

The impact of rectal surgery goes far beyond the physiological changes that in themselves are far reaching. The psychological trauma may induce social dysfunction, which will impact on all those within the patients' inner circle; however, with heightened awareness and sensitivity, all health care professionals can make a positive contribution to the rehabilitation process. An understanding of the underlying illness, treatment plan and potential complications is essential not only to make this contribution but also to ensure informed consent. Armed with the appropriate knowledge, skill and sensitivity, all health care professionals will help patients to make the transition from despair and despondency to adjustment and rehabilitation, enabling them to feel valued members of their families and society.

References

Audit Commission (1993) What Seems to be the Matter? Communication between hospitals and patients. London: HMSO.

Bailey CMH, Wheeler JMD, Birks M, Farouk RO (2003) The incidence and causes of permanent stoma after anterior resection. Colorectal Disease 5: 331.

Bond, CF (1997) Men and sexuality in stoma care. British Journal of Nursing 2(5): 260-263.

Borwell B (1997) The psychosexual needs of stoma patients. Professional Nurse 12(4) 250-255.

Burke M, Walsh M (1992) Gerontologic Nursing: Care of the frail elderly. Chicago: Mosby Year Book.

Burt K (1995) The effects of cancer on body image and sexuality. Nursing Times 91(7): 36-37.

Department of Health (1990) The Patient's Charter. London: HMSO.

Department of Health (1996) The Patient Partnership Strategy. London: HMSO.

Department of Health (1999) The Patient Partnership Strategy, 2nd edn. London: The Stationery Office.

Department of Health (2000) The NHS Plan: A plan for investment, A plan for reform. London: The Stationery Office.

Department of Health (2001a) Caring for Older People: A nursing priority. Integrating knowledge, practice and values. London: The Stationery Office.

Department of Health (2001b) The National Service Framework for Older People. London: The Stationery Office.

Department of Health (2002) Reference Guide to Consent for Examination or Treatment. London: The Stationery Office.

Devlin HB, Plant JA (1971) The aftermath of surgery for anorectal cancer. British Medical Journal 14: 413-418.

Dimond B (2001) Legal aspects of consent 3: nurses' duty of care to inform. British Journal of Nursing 10(7): 446-7.

Dimond B (2002) Legal aspects of consent 22: nurses' position when obtaining consent. British Journal of Nursing 11: 281-283.

Dorey G (2002) Outcome measures for erectile dysfunction 1: literature review. British Journal of Nursing 11(1): 54-63.

Fallowfield L, Ratcliffe D, Jenkins V, Saul J (2001) Psychiatric morbidity and its recognition by doctors in patients with cancer. British Journal of Cancer 84(8): 1011-1015.

Hargie O, McCartan PJ (1986) Social Skills Training and Psychiatric Nursing. London: Croom Helm.

Hughes A (1991) Life with a stoma. Nursing Times 87(25): 67-8.

Jacoby LH, Maloy B, Cirenza E, Shelton W, Goggins T, Balint J (1999) The basis for informed consent for bone marrow transplant patients. Bone Marrow Transplantation 23(7): 711-717

Kelman G, Minkler P (1985) An investigation of quality of life and self esteem among individuals with ostomies. Journal of Enterostomal Therapy 16: 4-11.

Kinrade S (2002) Communication breakdown. Nursing Times 98(3): 40-41.

Koshy KT (1989) I only have eyes for you. Nursing Times 85(30): 26-29.

Laurent C (1999) Aiding adjustment: how to help patients to adapt to life with a stoma. Nursing Times 95(30): 54-56.

McKee D (1999) The legal framework for informed consent. Professional Nurse 14(10): 688-90.

McKenzie F (1988) Sexuality after total pelvic exenteration. Nursing Times 84(20): 27-30.

Nursing and Midwifery Council (2002) Code of Professional Conduct: Protecting the public through professional standards. London: Nursing and Midwifery Council.

Pettitt E (1980) Body image. Nursing 16: 690-692.

Price B (1990) Body Image: Nursing concepts and care. London: Prentice Hall.

Salter M, Ziekenhuis C (1998) If you can help somebody ... (Nursing interventions to facilitate adaptation to an altered body image). Paper presented to the 12th Biennial Congress of the World Council of Enterostomal Therapists, Brighton.

Sanders T, Skevinton S (2003) Do bowel cancer patients participate? Treatment decision making. Findings from a qualitative study. European Journal of Cancer Care 12: 166.

Sprangers MAG, Taal BG, Aranson NK, te Velde A (1995) Quality of life in colorectal cancer: stoma v non stoma patients. Diseases of the Colon and Rectum 38: 361-369.

Taylor P (1994) Beating the taboo. Nursing Times 90: 1351-53.

Townley M (2002) Mental health needs of children and young people. Nursing Standard 16(30): 38-45.

Van Oijen E, Charnock A (1995) What is sexuality? Nursing Times 91(17): 26-27.

Walsh B (1995) Multidisciplinary management of altered body image. WOCN 22(5): 227-235.

Wallace B (2000) Nurses and consent. Professional Nurse 15: 11727-730.

Walshe K, Offen N (2001) A very public failure: lessons for quality improvement in healthcare organisations from Bristol Royal Infirmary. Quality in Health Care (10): 35-38.

White C (1998) Psychological management of stoma related concerns. Nursing Standard 12(36): 35-38.

White C, Unwin J (1998) Post-operative adjustment to surgery resulting in stoma: The importance of stoma-related cognitions. British Journal of Psychology 3: 85-93.

Chapter 7

Further treatment: chemotherapy and radiotherapy

Helen Ferns

Colorectal cancer is a common disease with approximately 33 000 new cases per annum in the UK (Office for National Statistics, 1998). The incidence of the disease is almost equal in men and women and rises sharply with age. It is rare below 40 years of age and 41 per cent of patients are over 75 (Office for National Statistics, 2000).

The management of colorectal cancer usually involves one of more of the following treatment modalities:

- Surgery
- Radiotherapy (predominately rectal cancer)
- Chemotherapy.

To achieve the best possible chance of cure, early diagnosis and appropriate surgical therapy are essential. Unfortunately, diagnosis is often delayed as a result of the vagueness of symptoms and a delayed realization of the significance of these symptoms (Ferns, 1999).

Survival is related to the spread of the disease at diagnosis (Table 7.1). Around 29 per cent of patients who present with colorectal cancer have distant metastases at the time of presentation (usually to the liver or lungs) (Smithies and Stein, 1999) and few of these patients will survive three years from the time of diagnosis (NHS Clinical Outcomes Group, 1997).

Table 7.1 Modified Dukes' staging of colorectal cancer, with 5-year survival

Dukes' stage (modified)	Definition	Frequency at diagnosis (%)	5-year survival rate (%)
A	Cancer localized to bowel wall	11	83
B	Cancer that penetrates the bowel wall	35	64
C	Cancer spread to the lymph nodes	26	38
D	Cancer with distant metastases	29	3

Source: Smithies and Stein (1999)

About 80 per cent of patients diagnosed with colorectal cancer undergo surgery (Effective Health Care, 1997). Many have potentially good survival outcomes after surgery, but over 50 per cent of those who have undergone surgery with apparently complete excision of the primary tumour will eventually relapse and die of the metastatic disease (Cunningham, 1996).

The most frequent site of metastatic disease is the liver. In as many as 30–40 per cent of patients with advanced disease, the liver may be the only site of spread, and for those patients surgery provides the only chance of cure. Reported 5-year survival rates for resection of liver metastasis range from 16 to 48 per cent (NHS Clinical Outcomes Group, 1997).

So what role does chemotherapy and radiotherapy play in the management of colorectal cancer? Adjuvant chemotherapy after potentially curative surgery for colon cancer and radiotherapy for rectal cancer reduce the incidence of recurrence and improve survival. In patients with advanced colorectal cancer, palliative chemotherapy improves the quality of life and increases survival (James, 1998).

This chapter gives an overview of the role of chemotherapy and radiotherapy in the management of colorectal cancer.

Radiotherapy

Radiotherapy is the use of ionizing radiation in the treatment of primarily malignant disease exerting local control over tumour tissue. Ionizing radiation destroys cells in the body by physical, chemical and biological methods. Radiation cannot distinguish between cancer and normal cells, so all cells within the treatment field are damaged, although cancer cells cannot repair radiation damage as effectively as normal cells. The aim of treatment is to deliver the required dose of radiation to the target area while minimizing the dose to the surrounding normal tissue. This is achieved by careful treatment planning to produce the best possible outcome in terms of survival, symptom relief and side effects. The treatment area must be accurately imaged so that the radiation beam can be accurately targeted; computed tomography (CT) facilitates precise delivery of radiotherapy to the treatment site, avoiding radiation of normal tissue. A multiple radiotherapy field technique is often used, bombarding the treatment area with multiple beams set to converge at a point deep within the treatment area, ensuring that the normal tissue receives minimal radiation. Different types of energy are required to treat different parts of the body; treatment fields close to the skin require less energy than treatment areas deep inside the body.

Radiation is measured in units called 'grays' (Gy) and the frequency in which it is given is referred to as 'fractionation'. Dosages are calculated to maintain a balance between killing any cancer cells without causing irreversible side effects to normal cells and tissue. Treatment is also dependent on whether the intent is to cure cancer at an early stage or at symptom relief in more advanced cancer. Radiotherapy can be delivered by various methods.

External beam radiotherapy

This is the most commonly used method of radiation treatment. The radiation beam is administered on to and into the patient from a source external to the patient's body. Treatment is delivered by high-energy X-ray machines known as linear accelerators. A course of treatment is prescribed, which can be anything from a single session to treatment lasting up to six weeks, depending on the site and stage performance status of the individual; it lasts about 2–3 minutes a day. The X-ray beam is accurately targeted by markings on the individual's skin or by the use of individually prepared Perspex shells.

Brachytherapy

Otherwise known as sealed source therapy, brachytherapy is a radioactive source placed within a body cavity or tissue or supported close to the skin surface. It was developed from the use of radium, but has largely been replaced by other radioisotopes, the properties of which make them less of a potential radiation hazard; it allows the radioactive sources to be remotely after-loaded into the tumour site, thus reducing the radiation hazard to individuals.

Liquid radioactive sources

Also known as unsealed source therapy, this is a radioactive substance delivered via injection or taken orally, the most common being radioactive iodine in the treatment of thyroid cancer.

Adjuvant radiotherapy for rectal cancer

In colon cancer there is no established role for adjuvant radiotherapy. Its goal in rectal cancer is to reduce the incidence of local recurrence, a potentially morbid complication. Local recurrence after complete resection of rectal cancer is more frequent than with colon cancer because the rectum lies below the peritoneal reflection. Of recurrences, 50 per cent are in the pelvis rather than at distant sites (Midgley and Kerr, 2001), and tumour invasion into the surrounding tissue and organs occurs more frequently because the growth of rectal tumours is not limited by a serosa (Ross and Cunningham, 1997).

Adjuvant radiotherapy has been evaluated for rectal cancer both before and after surgical resection.

Preoperative radiotherapy

A large number of randomized controlled trials (RCTs) have produced consistent evidence demonstrating that preoperative radiotherapy for rectal cancer reduces local recurrence rates (Association of Coloproctology of Great Britain and Ireland or ACPGB&I, 2001).

Mobile/Tethered/Operable tumours

Tumours that have not infiltrated surrounding structures are generally referred to as 'mobile/tethered tumours'. The objective of preoperative radiotherapy is to destroy micrometastatic disease and reduce the incidence of local recurrence. The Swedish rectal trial, which was the largest study of preoperative radiotherapy, demonstrated a reduction in local recurrence compared with surgery alone. Another Swedish study, the Uppsala trial, is the only reported trial that has directly compared pre- and postoperative radiotherapy, which also demonstrated a reduction in local recurrence rates after preoperative radiotherapy (Pahlman, 1998).

The schedule of radiotherapy is either a short-course 25 Gy over five days or long-course 45–50 Gy over 25 days. Where local imaging indicates a high risk of incomplete excision, long-course preoperative radiotherapy should be selected (ACPGB&I, 2001).

Recent improvements in the surgical excision of rectal cancers, e.g. total mesorectal excision (TME), has in some cases produced local recurrence rates as low as those seen in individuals treated with preoperative radiotherapy (McCall et al., 1995). However, preliminary results from a recent Dutch study have shown local recurrence rates of preoperative radiotherapy and TME surgery being further improved (Kapiteijn et al., 2001).

The Medical Research Council (MRC) CRO7 (MRC, 1998) trial, comparing preoperative radiotherapy and selective postoperative chemoradiation in rectal cancer, is hoping to address the question of radiotherapy in operable rectal cancer. The aim of the trial is to demonstrate whether preoperative short-course radiotherapy (25 Gy in five fractions), or optional postoperative radiotherapy (45–50 Gy in 25–30 fractions) to those individuals with a pathologically demonstrated high risk of recurrence, reduces the rate of local recurrence. The MRC CRO7 trial is currently still recruiting.

Postoperative radiotherapy

Postoperative, long-course, adjuvant radiotherapy reduces the incidences of local recurrence, but the benefit is less than that of preoperative radiotherapy. As with preoperative treatment, no benefit in overall survival has been demonstrated, although postoperative radiotherapy combined with 5-fluorouracil (5FU)-based chemotherapy demonstrates a significant survival advantage compared with surgery alone (Douglas et al., 1986; Krook et al., 1991). Postoperative chemoradiation is more commonly used in the USA; in European countries the tendency is to opt for preoperative short- or long-course radiotherapy, as previously described in operable tumours.

Individuals who have not had preoperative radiotherapy and shown postoperatively a high risk of tumour recurrence, with tumour involvement of the circumferential resection margin (CRM) or radial margins of < 1 mm clearance, should be considered for longer-course postoperative chemoradiation (ACGB&I, 2001).

Local recurrence rates are slightly improved when chemotherapy is combined with radiotherapy in the postoperative setting (Pahlman, 1998). The most common chemotherapy schedule is protracted venous infusion (PVI) of 5FU 200 mg/m^2 per day, on days 1–4 of weeks 1 and 5 of radiotherapy.

The toxicities of postoperative radiotherapy are significantly increased over preoperative treatment (Tepper et al., 1997), promoting the use of preoperative radiotherapy over postoperative in Europe.

Radiotherapy for locally advanced rectal cancer

Large numbers of individuals present with fixed rectal tumours, which have invaded surrounding structures and organs. To increase the resectability rate of fixed rectal tumours, preoperative radiotherapy is administered (Pahlam, 1998), at a dose of 45–50 Gy over 5 weeks, with the aim of producing tumour shrinkage. If possible, surgical resection takes place about 4–6 weeks later to allow for maximum tumour regression. The addition of chemotherapy is currently being evaluated in established trials.

For patients whose tumour dose not become amenable to surgical resection, the radiotherapy will, it is hoped, have provided some local control as well as symptomatic relief.

Radiotherapy for local regional recurrences

Preoperative chemoradiation has increased the resectability rates of locoregional recurrences (Rodel et al., 2000), but no evidence has been demonstrated in an RCT (Table 7.2). If recurrent disease is not amenable to surgical resection, chemoradiation can lead to an increase in symptomatic relief (ACPGB&I, 2001).

Table 7.2 Common chemoradiotherapy treatment schedules for rectal cancer

Treatment	Radiotherapy	Chemotherapy
Preoperative (short course)	25 Gy in 5 fractions	None
Preoperative (long course)	45-50 Gy in 25-30 fractions	None or PVI 5FU 200 mg/m^2/day on days 1-4 on first and last week of radiotherapy
Postoperative	45-50 Gy in 25-30 fractions	PVI 5FU 200mg/m^2 per day on days 1-4 first and last week of radiotherapy

5FU, 5-fluorouracil; PVI, protracted venous infusion

The toxicities of radiotherapy to the large bowel are common and cumulative; to be managed effectively, regular monitoring and intervention are essential throughout the treatment course.

The common side effects during treatment are:

- Bowels: alternating bowel actions, sensory alteration and abdominal cramps.
- Bladder: increase in micturition, urgency and burning sensation.
- Skin: red, dry, itchy and sometimes broken down if tumour is low down in the rectum, resulting in a higher dose of radiation to the anal skin area.
- Fatigue: cumulative throughout the treatment, usually peaking the week after completion of radiotherapy and taking up to 6-8 weeks to resolve.

Long-term/Permanent side effects:
- Menopause: in females
- Reduced sperm count in males
- Permanent damage to the bladder or bowel.

Palliative radiotherapy for advanced colorectal cancer

Palliative radiotherapy is usually given for the relief of symptoms of advanced disease. The treatment of distant metastases, such as lung, brain and bone as well as the pelvic recurrences, with either single fraction or short courses of radiotherapy can lead to a symptomatic benefit. The aim of palliative radiotherapy is to obtain a balance between symptom management and treatment toxicities. Treatment is dependent on the individual's performance status (Table 7.3), volume of disease and previous radiotherapy.

Table 7.3 World Health Organization (WHO) performance status

WHO grade	Characteristics
0	Able to carry out all normal activity without restriction
1	Restricted in physically strenuous activity but ambulatory and able to carry out light work
2	Ambulatory and capable of all self-care but unable to carry out any work; up and about more than 50% of waking hours
3	Capable only of limited self-care; confined to bed or chair more than 50% of waking hours
4	Completely disabled; cannot carry out any self-care; totally confined to bed or chair

Source: WHO (1979)

Chemotherapy

Chemotherapy was developed in the 1940s. Chemotherapy drugs used in the treatment of cancer are referred to as cytotoxic agents: 'cyto' means 'cell', and 'toxic' means 'poison'.

Cytotoxic drugs can broadly be grouped into classes relating to their anti-tumour action at cell level. Mode of action depends on the individual drug, but most drugs in current use inhibit cellular proliferation, by inhibiting DNA or RNA synthesis. The primary classification of cytotoxic drugs is according to their action on the cell life cycle, those that are cell cycle specific (CCPS) or active in all phases of the cell cycle, and those that are cell cycle phase non-specific (CCPNS) or active in specific phases (Weinstein, 1993). Further conventional classification of cytotoxic agents is by their biochemical mechanisms of action on the cell, those with similar modes of action being grouped together.

Alkylating agents

These exert their main toxicity by forming cross-linkages between DNA chains, which result in the inhibition of DNA replication and subsequent cell division; also by interacting with a number of enzymes involved in protein synthesis, they prevent DNA synthesis and cell division, e.g. cyclophosphamide or oxaliplatin.

Antimetabolites

These interfere with the production of purine and pyrimidine and thus prevent protein synthesis. They inhibit enzymes, or become incorporated in new nuclear material altering function, e.g. methotrexate, 5-fluorouracil, capecitabine, UFT.

Cytotoxic antibiotics

These are divided into anthracyclines or non-anthracyclines. Anthracyclines intercalate between DNA base-pairs, inhibiting DNA and RNA synthesis, and also producing free radicals that can break the DNA chain. Both have an alkylating activity and affect permeability of the cell membrane, e.g. doxorubicin.

Mitotic spindle inhibitors

These bind to the protein of cellular microtubles known as tubulin, inhibiting spindle formation and causing metaphase arrest, which leads to the disruption of cell division, e.g. vincristine.

Topoisomerase I inhibitors

These are S phase specific, inhibiting the action of topoisomerase I, an enzyme that releases the torsional strain in the supercoiled DNA by catalysing a transient break in one of its strands, allowing replication to take place. They act by stabilizing the cleavable complex formed between the enzyme and DNA strand and, as a result, the cleavable complex does not dissociate and the repair of the strand is prevented, resulting in cessation of the advancement of the replication fork, e.g. irinotecan.

Taxoids/Taxanes

These work by arresting cell division during the metaphase of the cell cycle. As the spindle forms during mitosis, the taxoids/taxanes promote the assembly of the microtubules but then stop their disassembly by inhibiting the depolymerization of the contractile protein tubulin. As a result, the microtubular network becomes abnormally rigid and unable to perform vital mitotic and interphase cellular functions, which eventually leads to cell death, e.g. paclitaxel (Taxol).

Miscellaneous agents

These work by various ways of inhibiting cell proliferation.

Cytotoxic drugs can be administered by a variety of routes: oral, intra-muscular, intravenous, intra-arterial and intravesicular. All are blood borne and have the potential to treat both primary and metastatic disease. As cytotoxic drugs cannot differentiate between cancer and normal cells, they affect all cells. The cells most affected are the rapidly proliferating cells of the mouth, gastrointestinal tract, bone marrow and hair follicles. This is why side effects in these areas are generally more severe.

Adjuvant chemotherapy for colorectal cancer (Table 7.4)

Adjuvant is derived from the Latin 'ad' meaning 'to' and 'juvare' mean-ing 'help'.

The rationale for adjuvant treatment is the failure of surgery to cure, probably as a result of microscopic tumour cells that have metastasized before primary tumour resection and which are undetectable by radio-logical investigation. The aim of adjuvant treatment is to target rapidly cycling foci of cancer cells and destroy them before they become estab-lished detectable metastasis (Midgley and Kerr, 1998).

Until the late 1980s, the role of adjuvant chemotherapy in colorectal cancer was unclear. Studies published in 1989 and 1990 showed, for the first time, the clinical benefit of 5FU in the adjuvant setting (Laurie et al., 1989; Moertel et al., 1990).

5-Fluorouracil is a cell-cycle-specific agent, active during one short phase of the cell life. It is a thymidylate synthetase (TS) inhibitor that pre-vents formation of thymidine, inhibiting DNA and RNA synthesis. The addition of folinic acid (FA) stabilizes the 5FU–TS complex, promoting and maximizing TS inhibition.

Recent results from large randomized phase III trials have demonstrat-ed a moderate increase in disease-free survival at three years and overall survival for individuals with Dukes' C colon cancer treated with a sys-temic combination chemotherapy of 5FU and FA (Midgley and Kerr, 2001) – a 6 per cent increase in the 5-year survival rate or prevention of six deaths per 100 individuals treated with adjuvant chemotherapy (NHS Clinical Outcome Group, 1997). As large numbers of individuals are diagnosed with colorectal cancer, the place for adjuvant chemotherapy is justified.

Current evidence therefore suggests that a combination of 5FU and FA should be accepted as standard adjuvant chemotherapy for individuals with resected Dukes' C colon cancer (Midgely and Kerr, 2001).

Table 7.4 Common adjuvant chemotherapy regimens for colon cancer

Regimen	Dosing	Schedule	Toxicities
Weekly bolus 'Quasar' schedule	FA 20 mg/m^2 intravenous bolus 5FU 375 mg/m^2 intravenous bolus	Weekly for 30 weeks	Mucositis, neutropenia, nausea and vomiting, diarrhoea, hand and foot syndrome, and fatigue
Mayo Clinic	FA 20 mg/m^2 intravenous bolus 5FU 425 mg/m^2 intravenous bolus	Daily for 5 consecutive days Repeated every 4 weeks for 6 cycles	Mucositis, neutropenia, nausea and vomiting, diarrhoea, hand and foot syndrome, and fatigue
Roswell Park	FA 500 mg/m^2 intravenous over 2 h 5FU 500 mg/m^2 intravenous bolus 1 h after FA infusion started	Weekly for 6 weeks Repeated every 8 weeks for 4 cycles	Mucositis, neutropenia, nausea and vomiting, diarrhoea, hand and foot syndrome, and fatigue

FA, folinic acid; 5FU, 5-fluorouracil.

The grade of side effects varies for each of the above regimens, with the weekly bolus regimen, which is more commonly used in the UK, generally being the least toxic.

The question of duration of treatment has been evaluated in a North American Study comparing six months of treatment against 12 months of treatment. Results have demonstrated that six months is as effective as 12 months (Midgely and Kerr, 1998), with positive quality-of-life and financial implications in health care provision. The optimal dosing regimen of FA has also been widely evaluated, because high-dose FA is 10 times more expensive than low-dose FA. In the United Kingdom Co-ordinating Committee on Cancer Research (UKCCCR), Quasar Study (Quick, Simple and Reliable), the certain arm indication has demonstrated no survival advantage of high-dose versus low-dose FA (Midgely and Kerr, 2001).

Although the evidence for the use of adjuvant chemotherapy in resected Dukes' C colorectal cancer is clear, there is less evidence for its use in resected Dukes' B tumours, even though this group of individuals is more frequently being offered treatment. The uncertain arm of the Quasar Study (Quasar 1 – a UKCCCR study of adjuvant chemotherapy for colorectal cancer) is aiming to establish whether adjuvant chemotherapy is justified in Dukes' B colorectal cancer and to illustrate which factors might help demonstrate chemotherapeutic benefit. Randomization is between treatment and no treatment for individuals with an uncertain indication for adjuvant chemotherapy. Recruitment has yet to be completed. The controversy is not whether adjuvant chemotherapy is effective in resected Dukes' B colorectal cancer, but rather the absolute increase in cure rate with treatment. The decision to use adjuvant chemotherapy in resected Dukes' B colorectal cancer must be individualized; recruitment into current clinical trials must be considered as well as tumour differentiation, and adjacent structure and organ invasion or tumour perforation should be considered.

For Dukes' B or C rectal cancer, there is inadequate randomized research evidence to assess the benefit of adjuvant chemotherapy. Recent adjuvant studies have been limited to individuals with colon cancer. The best estimate of the effect of 5FU/FA adjuvant chemotherapy in rectal cancer is therefore about the same as for colon cancer (NHS Clinical Outcomes Group, 1997) and recruitment into ongoing clinical trials is advised.

It is assumed that the earlier adjuvant chemotherapy is commenced after resection of the primary tumour the greater the potential benefit, although there is no clinical evidence to illustrate this (Midgely and Kerr, 2001). Current standards within the UK recommend starting chemotherapy within eight weeks of curative surgical resection.

Palliative chemotherapy for advanced colorectal cancer

For individuals with advanced colorectal cancer, chemotherapy is administered with palliative rather than curative intent. Advanced colorectal cancer has been defined as colorectal cancer that, at presentation or recurrence, is either metastatic or so locally advanced that surgical resection is unlikely to be carried out with curative intent (Young and Rea, 2001).

Palliative chemotherapy is now offered to an increasing proportion of patients with advanced colorectal cancer; the aims of chemotherapy in this group of patients is to prolong survival, control symptoms, and maintain or improve quality of life (Seymour et al., 1997).

The selection of individuals for palliative chemotherapy requires the opinion of an oncologist experienced in the treatment of colorectal cancer. Poor performance status (3 or 4), low serum albumin, high alkaline phosphatase and liver involvement are independent predictors of progression, and low serum albumin, high glutamyl transferase and high carcinoembryonic antigen (CEA) are predictors for poor survival (Fontzilas et al., 1996).

The potential benefits of chemotherapy in the palliative setting must be weighed against any potential treatment toxicities and effect on quality of life. The continuing assessment of treatment-related side effects and correct management is essential in determining the acceptability of chemotherapy in the palliative setting.

5FU has been the only active drug available in the management of colorectal cancer for the past 40 years. A combination of 5FU with a biochemical modulator such as FA has been the standard treatment for advanced colorectal cancer, increasing survival by about 3–6 months, as well as improving symptom control, performance status (see Table 7.3) and quality of life (Scheithauer et al., 1993).

Controversy exists around the world as to the optimal 5FU regimen; it is an important issue when evaluating the results of clinical trials conducted with various 5FU regimens as the standard arm (Cassidy, 2001).

Current evidence, however, suggests that 5FU administered in an infusional form (of at least 24 hours' duration) doubles response rate, increases median survival and reduces toxicity over bolus regimens (Meta-Analysis Group in Cancer, 1998). Infusional regimens are accepted as standard therapy in Europe and should therefore be used as standard therapy over bolus regimens for advanced colorectal cancer (Table 7.5).

Table 7.5 Infusional 5FU regimens for the treatment of advanced colorectal cancer

Regimen	Method of administration	Common side effects
deGramont (5FU/FA)	Infused over 48 hours every 2 weeks (usually requires indwelling central or peripheral line)	Mucositis, neutropenia, nausea and vomiting, diarrhoea, hand and foot syndrome, and fatigue
Lokich (5FU)	Continuous infusion (requires ambulatory pump and indwelling central or peripheral line)	Mucositis, neutropenia, nausea and vomiting, diarrhoea, hand and foot syndrome, and fatigue

Source: NHS Clinical Outcomes Group (1997)

The toxicities of infusional 5FU with or without FA are usually manageable and both regimens are well tolerated, with minimal disruption of functional status. Education of individuals about the common side effects and prompt management can, however, reduce grade of toxicity. Both regimens require an indwelling central or peripheral line and individuals must be made aware of any limitations of living with an indwelling line and the potential complications.

Current evidence indicates that the start of early chemotherapy before clinical deterioration for advanced disease can improve the response rate of treatment and overall survival by 3–6 months without any adverse effect on quality of life (Scheithauer et al., 1993).

There is much debate about the optimum duration of chemotherapy; common practice is to vary between 12 and 24 weeks or until disease progression. A recent study, which compared two different durations of chemotherapy (12 or 24 weeks) in patients with stable or responding disease, has suggested that 12 weeks of treatment, with close observation until disease progression, is not detrimental to survival and contributes towards quality of life (Maughan et al., 2001).

In recent years the availability of several new agents with different mechanisms of action has shown improved activity in the treatment of advanced colorectal cancer, both in chemotherapy-naïve individuals and in those with disease refractory to 5FU.

Irinotecan

Irinotecan represents a novel class of cytotoxic drug, the camptothecins. The active component of irinotecan is a selective inhibitor of topoisomerase I, an enzyme that plays a pivotal role in DNA transcription, replication and repair, leading to multiple single-strand DNA breaks, which eventually block the replication fork, leading to cell death.

Colorectal cancer cells have high levels of the enzyme topoisomerase I; irinotecan's, inhibition of this enzyme explains its activity in colorectal cancer. Multiple RCTs with irinotecan have shown a survival benefit in individuals with advanced colorectal cancer (Cunningham et al., 1998; Rougier et al., 1998; Douillard et al., 2000; Saltz et al., 2000).

Indications for treatment are first-line combination with 5FU/FA in individuals who have had no prior chemotherapy for advanced disease and as second-line single agent in individuals who have progressed after an established 5FU regimen.

First-line combination treatment is administered for 48 hours via a centrally placed line, either a Hickman or a peripherally inserted central catheter (PICC), every 14 days for a total of six cycles before assessment of tumour response. Second-line treatment with irinotecan is given as a single agent. Treatment is administered via an intravenous infusion lasting between 30 and 60 minutes, every 21 days for four cycles before assessment of tumour response.

The side effects of irinotecan are generally manageable and non-cumulative; the severity of toxicity is usually increased in the second-line single agent therapy.

Acute cholinergic syndrome

This usually occurs within 24 hours of treatment administration; it is short lasting, but never life threatening, and is very unpleasant for the patient, treatable and preventable, and should never lead to treatment discontinuation. Treatment is by a subcutaneous injection of atropine sulphate 0.25 mg and is then given prophylactically before each administration.

Early diarrhoea

This is diarrhoea that occurs in the first 24 hours of treatment administration; treatment should be with atropine, because this is related to the acute cholinergic syndrome.

Nausea and vomiting

These can occur concurrently after each administration of treatment. It is usually controllable with effective antiemetic therapy, which is commonly administered intravenously before each cycle, with oral treatment being given to take home as required

Delayed diarrhoea

This is diarrhoea that usually occurs more than 24 hours after treatment administration. It is predictable at around 5 days and is usually short-lived, lasting about 12–72 hours. Delayed diarrhoea is the most common dose-limiting toxicity of irinotecan therapy.

Neutropenia

This is the second most dose-limiting toxicity; it rarely develops into febrile neutropenia and is non-cumulative. The median day to nadir is 8 days.

Once again, the incidence of the grade of neutropenia is different between first-line combination treatment and second-line single-agent treatment. The severity in combination treatment is less.

Alopecia

This is more common when irinotecan is administered as a single agent; incidence and grade are reduced when given in combination with 5FU/FA

Although all patients should be prepared for some hair loss, it occurs gradually as the cycles continue and hair loss is reversed when treatment is discontinued.

Oxaliplatin

Oxaliplatin is a new platinum derivative analogue and is a potent inhibitor of DNA synthesis. It is thought to act as an alkylating agent, making DNA lesions that the cell cannot repair and leading to cell death (Cvitkovic and Betradda, 1999). It shows synergism with 5FU.

Several RCTs have demonstrated that oxaliplatin added to the 5FU/FA regimen shows an improved response rate and time to progression, but there is no difference in overall survival. One study demonstrated an increased number of individuals undergoing potential curative surgical resection of liver metastasis (Giacchetti et al., 2000).

Oxiplatin is licensed for use in the UK for the first-line treatment of advanced colorectal cancer in combination with 5FU/FA. First-line combination treatment is administered for 48 hours via a centrally placed line, either a Hickman or a PICC, every 14 days for a total of six cycles before assessment of tumour response.

The side effects of oxaliplatin are generally manageable and, apart from neurotoxicity, they are non-cumulative.

Sensory peripheral neurotoxicity
This is the most distinguishable side effect of oxaliplatin treatment. If symptoms have not resolved between each cycle and there is a loss of function (fine finger control), oxaliplatin should be stopped until the sensory neuropathy has resolved.

Pharyngeal dysaesthesia
Otherwise known as 'funny throat syndrome', this is precipitated by cold and can cause considerable distress to an individual if not he or she is reassured about it.

Renal function
Oxaliplatin is not nephrotoxic but is renally cleared. Renal function should be monitored before treatment administration.

Hair thinning
Alopecia is uncommon but as treatment cycles continue individuals might notice a thinning of hair.

Nausea and vomiting
These can occur concurrently after each administration of treatment. It is usually controllable with effective antiemetic therapy, which is usually administered intravenously before each cycle, and oral treatment is given to take home as required.

Raltitrexed

Raltitrexed is a selective TS inhibitor. It is licensed in the UK for the palliative treatment of colorectal cancer for patients in whom 5FU is not tolerated or is inappropriate. It is a convenient 15-min infusion every three weeks and, although evidence suggests survival data comparable with 5FU, toxicity is unpredictable as highlighted in the MRC CRO6 trial, which reported an increase in the toxic death rate (Maughan et al., 2001).

Common toxicities associated with raltitrexed are diarrhoea, nausea and vomiting, myelosuppression and increased liver transaminases.

Capecitabine

Capecitabine is the first of a new class of oral fluoropyrimidines, a pro-drug of 5FU. It was designed to mimic continuous infusion 5FU and to generate 5FU preferentially in tumour tissue. The tumour-selective activity of capecitabine is achieved through the exploitation of the high concentrations of thymidine phosphorylase (TP) present in colorectal cancer cells compared with normal cells.

Two RCTs have demonstrated that, in advanced colorectal cancer, capecitabine shows a significantly better response rate, equivalent time to progression, and overall survival when compared with a bolus regimen of 5FU/FA (Hoff, 2000). Capecitabine was also less toxic in most respects and more convenient to administer. It is licensed for use in advanced colorectal cancer.

Capecitabine is taken twice daily in equally divided doses for 14 days followed by a rest period for seven days.

The most common side effects of capecitabine are similar to those of 5FU; incidence and grade of toxicity vary between individuals and 5FU regimen.

Hand and foot syndrome
This is one of the most commonly reported toxicities and, depending on the grade, can lead to dose reduction.

Diarrhoea, stomatitis, nausea and vomiting, and alopecia
These are also common toxicities and are managed continuously as per local guidelines. As always, the grade of toxicity has to be effectively monitored to gain maximum benefits from treatment and defer or dose reduce as appropriate.

UFT

Ftorafur is another oral pro-drug of 5FU that has been around since the 1960s. Uracil is added to ftorafur to form UFT, which acts as a competitor for the rate-limiting enzyme in the catabolic inactivation of 5FU, which extends the plasma half-life of 5FU.

Two RCTs have demonstrated that UFT/FA was equivocal in response rate, time to progression and overall survival when compared with bolus 5FU/FA; it is generally better tolerated and more convenient to administer (Carmichael et al., 1999; Pazdur et al., 1999). UFT is licensed for use in advanced colorectal cancer.

Hand and foot syndrome diarrhoea, stomatitis, nausea and vomiting, and alopecia
These are also common toxicities and are managed continuously as per local guidelines. As always, the grade of toxicity has to be effectively monitored to gain maximum benefits from treatment and defer or dose reduce as appropriate.

Fatigue
Fatigue is a commonly reported problem experienced by many individuals during treatment for cancer. It is frustrating and overwhelming and can have a serious impact on an individual's quality of life. All treatments used in the management of bowel cancer can induce fatigue and, when mutimodality treatments are delivered, the effect of fatigue can be intensified. All nurses and health-care professionals involved in the care and treatment of individuals with bowel cancer must be aware of the signs and symptoms of fatigue and support the individual in a strategy of management or coping with this common and debilitating complaint.

5-Fluorouracil/FA is still the mainstay of treatment for metastatic colorectal cancer. Newer agents are rightly gaining a place in the first- and second-line treatment of advanced colorectal cancer, some showing an improvement in progression-free survival, and in the case of irinotecan, overall improvement in survival (Young and Rea, 2001). Optimum sequencing and combination of 5FU/FA, irinotecan and oxaliplatin are the subject of an ongoing trial, the MRC CRO8 (FOCUS; MRC, 2001), which is currently recruiting in the UK.

Chemotherapy prolongs the time to tumour progression and the overall survival of individuals with advanced colorectal cancer. Even though chemotherapy is potentially toxic, the increase in overall survival and the palliative benefits make them more acceptable. There is mounting evidence that all individuals with advanced colorectal cancer should be offered chemotherapy, depending on physical functioning. Individuals should be allowed to make informed decisions, balancing the relatively small gains in overall survival and improvement in quality of life against the potential treatment toxicities (Michael and Zalcberg, 2000).

The future

In recent years new cytotoxic agents have become available for the treatment of colorectal cancer; it is hoped that during the next few years we shall see the use of different combinations of these agents in both the adjuvant and the palliative setting, improving survival and maximizing quality of life. But will this result in dramatic increase in the 5-year survival rate?

Possibly the future lies in a different direction; early phase I studies are already under way looking at signal transduction modulators, anti-angiogenic agents and gene therapy.

Anal cancer

Cancer of the anal region accounts for 3–3.5 per cent of all colorectal tumours. Peak incidence is between 58 and 64 years. The distribution of incidence has changed since the 1960s, with a particular increase in incidence among young men and older women.

Most patients are treated with multimodality therapy. Up until the late 1980s, surgery was the predominant treatment of choice for anal cancer within the UK. But in more recent years the non-surgical management with radiotherapy or combined radiotherapy and chemotherapy has resulted in comparable survival rates without the need for colostomy (UKCCCR Anal Cancer Working Party, 1996).

Retrospective studies comparing the use of radiotherapy alone and combined radiotherapy and chemotherapy have demonstrated that combined therapy had a higher primary control rate (Cummings, 1992).

Chemoradiation is now regarded as the primary intervention for anal cancer in the UK (Osbourne et al., 2001), with a reduction in the need for colostomy formation in this patient group. Abdominoperineal resection is usually left in reserve for local recurrences.

Radiotherapy is given over 4–5 weeks with a boost given either as an implant or an external beam after a break of up to six weeks. Concurrent chemotherapy is administered at weeks 1 and 4–5 of radiotherapy – a combination of infusional 5FU and either mitomycin or cisplatin.

After the publication of several studies from various institutions, a continuous course of radiotherapy has been recommended; rather than having a delay of up to six weeks, boost treatment is delivered immediately after the scheduled radiotherapy by external beam (UKCCCR Anal Cancer Working Party, 2001).

The UKCCCR Anal Cancer Working Party launched the ACT II Anal Cancer Trial in 2001. The main objectives of the study are to evaluate whether cisplatin given concurrently with 5FU and radiotherapy produces a higher complete remission rate than mitomycin C, plus whether maintenance chemotherapy after chemoradiation will improve recurrence-free survival by preventing or delaying disease dissemination (UKCCCR Anal Cancer Working Party, 2001).

Toxicities can be very severe in combined treatment schedules, and individuals require support and education to manage and cope with side effects effectively. Moist desquamation of the perianal and surrounding skin is common, and intensive symptom control is required.

Oncology team

The management of patients with colorectal cancer is multifaceted, including treatment, symptom management, and emotional and psychosocial support.

The multidisciplinary team encompasses oncologist, radiographers, chemotherapy nurse, specialist nurses, trials team, dieticians, medical social worker and rehabilitation team.

Radiotherapy treatment is generally delivered in large cancer centres/units that have the expertise in the safe management of individuals undergoing radiotherapy.

Chemotherapy should be administered in designated units that specialize in the administration of cytotoxic chemotherapy, and be supervised by a suitably trained oncologist.

Specialist oncology teams are used to managing the unwanted side effects of chemotherapy/radiotherapy and maximizing the benefits of treatment. Education of the individual receiving chemotherapy about management of potential toxicities is essential. Oral and written information must be provided, with a 24-hour contact number. Also, education of the staff involved ensures that the incidence and severity of side effects are minimized. Local standard management guidelines have usually been developed to promote good practice and quality patient care.

The pathway of care for an individual with colorectal cancer is continually moving among primary, secondary and tertiary care settings; increased communication and the sharing of information can only improve the whole package of care to the individual, resulting in improved outcomes.

With the increased used of ambulatory chemotherapy in advanced colorectal cancer, increased links have been established with the primary health-care team, who can be responsible for the disconnection of infusers and the care of central and peripheral lines. The oncology team must ensure that district nurses are kept up to date in the management of individuals receiving ambulatory chemotherapy, using local guidelines, as well as providing support and advice.

Over recent years, individuals with advanced colorectal cancer have seen an increase in overall survival, with the use of palliative chemotherapy and the availability of new agents. But that survival is on average about 18 months, so liaison with local palliative care teams is advisable early on, to ensure good palliation of symptoms and psychosocial support.

Implications for nurses

The cure/care dichotomy in advanced colorectal cancer must fall on the side of individual care and optimal quality of life. Patients and families, nurses and other health professionals share an interest in maximizing positive outcomes by making the best decisions for the welfare of the patient.

The oncology nurse is in an ideal position to help the individual obtain information about various treatment options in order to make an informed choice and give consent. High priority is given to individual autonomy in our society, and many ethical questions arise as practical matters as a result of the values placed on this concept, e.g. this is the moral basis for obtaining informed consent as well as for accepting informed refusal, respecting the individual's right to make decisions. For individuals to give informed consent, they must be able to decide whether the likelihood of longer life is worth the additional morbidity caused by treatment. Information on quality of life outcomes can assist in the decision-making process.

There is evidence of significant variation in the process and outcomes of colorectal cancer nationally and internationally. Current guidelines advocate the use of chemotherapy in advanced and recurrent disease; whether the decision is to treat or to palliate in order to extend life in advanced/recurrent disease, quality-of-life issues should be the main focus.

Quality of life in cancer care is increasingly recognized as a valuable supplement to tumour response and survival data, providing the individual a perspective on therapies and a way of evaluating whether small gains in life span come at too high a cost. Taking into account the individual's assessment of quality of life during treatment might give a different perception of toxicity and efficacy from that of the clinician.

Conclusion

Colorectal cancer has a major health impact on the population of the UK. Treatments can be complicated and have a major impact on the quality and length of an individual's life. The use of combination treatments in both the adjuvant and the palliative setting can, it is hoped, improve survival rates and extend life.

Although 50 per cent of patients with bowel cancer can expect to be cured with surgery, 50 per cent go on to develop metastatic disease. Historically, treatment options have been limited for this group of individuals. The development and availability of new treatment options offer encouragement and extend the range of options available to oncologists.

It is vital for individuals and oncologists to have a choice when considering treatment for advanced bowel cancer, because no single treatment will be suitable for all individuals, when balancing stage of disease, treatment responses and quality of life.

References

Association of Coloproctology of Great Britain and Ireland (2001) Guidelines for the Management of Colorectal Cancer. London: Royal College of Surgeons.

Cassidy J (2001) Reports of Colorectal Cancer. Colorectal Cancer Forum E-bulletin. Succinct Communications.

Carmichael J et al. (1999) Randomised comparative study of ORZEL plus leucovorin versus parental 5FU plus leucovorin in patients with metastatic colorectal cancer. Proceedings of the American Society of Clinical Oncologists 18: 264a (abstract 1015).

Cummings BJ (1992) Concomitant XRT and chemotherapy for anal cancer. Journal of Oncology 19(suppl 11): 102-108.

Cunningham D (1996) Current status of colorectal cancer: cpt11 (irinotecan) a therapeutic innovation. European Journal of Cancer 32A(suppl 3): S1-S8.

Cunningham D, Pyrhonen S, James RD et al. (1998) Randomised trial of irinotecan plus supportive care vs supportive care alone after fluorouracil failure for patients with metastatic colorectal cancer. The Lancet 352: 1413-1418

Cvikovic E, Betradda M (1999) Oxaliplatin: A new therapeutic option in colorectal cancer. Seminars in Oncology 26: 647-662.

Douillard JY, Cunningham D, Roth AD et al. (2000) Irinotecan combined with fluorouracil compared with fluorouracil alone as first line treatment for metastatic colorectal cancer: a multicentre randomised trial. The Lancet 335: 1041-1047.

Douglas HO Jr, Moertel CG, Mayer RJ et al. (1986) Survival after postoperative combination treatment of rectal cancer. New England Journal of Medicine 315: 1294-1295.

Effective Health Care (1997). The Management of Colorectal Cancer. NHS Centre for Reviews and Dissemination, University of York.

Ferns H (1999) Campto: effective chemotherapy for advanced colorectal cancer. International Journal of Palliative Nurses 5(6):

Fontzilas G, Gossios K, Zisiadis A et al. (1996) A prognostic variable in patients with advanced colorectal cancer treated with fluorouracil and leucovorin-based chemotherapy. Medical and Paediatric Oncology 26: 305-317.

Giacchetti S, Perpoint B, Zidani R et al. (2000) Phase III multicentre randomised trial of oxaliplatin added to chronomodulated fluorouracil-leucovorin as first line treatment of metastatic colorectal cancer. Journal of Clinical Oncology 18: 136-147.

Hoff PM (2000) Capecitabine as first-line treatment for colorectal cancer: integrated results of 1207 patients from a randomised phase III studies. Annals of Oncology 11(suppl 4): 62 (abstract 271).

James RD (1998) First line therapy: new medical evidence from ongoing trials. In: Cunningham D, Allen-Marsh T, Miles A (eds), The Effective Management of Metastatic Colorectal Cancer. London: Aesculapius Medical Press, pp. 35-53.

Kapiteijn JNE et al. (2001) Pre-operative radiotherapy combined with TME for resectable rectal cancer. New England Journal of Medicine 345: 638-646.

Krook JE, Moertel CG, Gunderson LL et al. (1991) Effective surgical adjuvant for high risk rectal carcinoma. New England Journal of Medicine 324: 709–715.

Laurie JA, Moertel CG, Fleming TR et al. (1989) Surgical adjuvant therapy of large bowel carcinoma: an evaluation of levamisole and the combination of levamisole and 5-fluorouracil. Journal of Clinical Oncology 1989: 1447–1456.

McCall JL, Cox MR, Wattchow DA (1995) Analysis of local recurrence rate after surgery alone for rectal cancer. International Colorectal Disease 10: 126–133.

Maughan TS, James RD, Kerr D et al. (1999) Preliminary results of multi-randomised trial comparing 3 chemotherapy regimens (deGramont, Lokich and Ralitrexed) in metastatic colorectal cancer. American Society of Clinical Oncologists on-line 1007

Maughan TS, James RD, Kerr D et al. (2001) Continuous versus intermittent chemotherapy for advanced colorectal cancer: preliminary results of MRC CRO6b randomisation trial. Proceedings of the American Society of Clinical Oncologists 20: 125a.

Medical Research Council (1997) Trial Protocol CRO6 – Chemotherapy choices in advanced colorectal cancer. A randomised trial comparing 2 durations and 3 systemic chemotherapy regimens in the palliative treatment of advanced colorectal cancer. London: MRC Trials Office.

Medical Research Council (1998) Trial Protocol CRO7 – A randomised trial comparing pre-operative radiotherapy and selective post-operative chemoradiotherapy in rectal cancer. London: MRC Trials Office.

Medical Research Council (2001) Trial Protocol CRO8 – A randomised trial to assess the role of irinotecan and oxaliplatin in advanced colorectal cancer. London: MRC Trials Office.

Meta-Analysis Group in Cancer (1998) Efficacy of intravenous continuous infusion of fluorouracil compared with bolus administration in advanced colorectal cancer. Journal of Clinical Oncology 16: 301–308.

Michael M, Zalcberg JR (eds) (2000) Palliative chemotherapy for advanced colorectal cancer: systematic review and meta-analysis. British Medical Journal 321: 531–535.

Midgley R, Kerr D (1998) Systemic adjuvant therapy of colon cancer. In: Bleiberg H, Rougier P, Wilke H (eds), Management of Colorectal Cancer. London: Martin Dunitz.

Midgley R, Kerr D (2001) In: Kerr D, Young A, Hobbs R (eds), ABC of Colorectal Cancer. London: BMJ Books

Moertel CG, Fleming TR, Macdonald JS et al. (1990) Levamisole and fluorouracil for adjuvant therapy of resected colon carcinoma. New England Journal of Medicine 322: 352–358.

NHS Clinical Outcomes Group (1997) Guidance on Commissioning Cancer Services, Improving Outcomes in Colorectal Cancer. London: Department of Health.

Office for National Statistics (1998) Cancer Registry. London: HMSO.

Office for National Statistics (2000) Mortality Statistics. London: HMSO.

Osbourne M, Glynne-Jones R, Makris A (2001) Chemoradiation followed by immediate boost in squamous cell carcinoma of the anus. Proceedings of the American Society of Clinical Oncologists.

Pahlman L (1998) Preoperative treatment of rectal cancer. In: Bleiberg H, Rougier P, Wilke H (eds), Management of Colorectal Cancer. London: Martin Dunitz.

Pazdur R et al. (1999) Multi-centre phase III study of 5-FU or UFT in combination with leucovorin in patients with metastatic colorectal cancer. Proceedings of the American Society of Clinical Oncologists 18: 263a (abstract 1009).

Rodel C, Grabenhauer GG, Matzel KE et al. (2000) Extensive surgery after high-dose pre-operative chemoradiotherapy for locally advanced recurrent colorectal cancer. Diseases of the Colon and Rectum 43: 312–319.

Ross P, Cunningham (1997) Colorectal Cancer. The National Association of Fundholding Practices. Official Yearbook 1997–98.

Rougier P, Van Cutsem E, Bajetta E et al. (1998) Randomised trial of irinotecan vs fluorouracil by continuous infusion after fluorouracil failure in patients with metastatic colorectal cancer. The Lancet 352: 1407–1412.

Saltz LB, Cox JV, Blanke C et al. (2000) Irinotecan plus fluorouracil and leucovorin for metastatic colorectal cancer. Irinotecan Study Group. New England Journal of Medicine 343: 905-914.

Scheithauer W, Rosen J, Kornek GV, Sebesta C, Depisch D (1993) Randomised comparison of combination chemotherapy plus supportive care with supportive care alone in patients with metastatic CRC. British Medical Journal 306: 752-755.

Seymour MT, Stenning SP, Cassidy J (1997) Attitudes and practice in the management of metastatic colorectal in Britain. Colorectal Cancer Working Party of the UK MRC. Clinical Oncology 9: 248-251.

Smithies A, Stein K (1999) Irinotecan as second line chemotherapy in colorectal cancer (Dec report; no. 97). University of Southampton, Wessex Institute for Health Research and Development.

Tepper JE, O'Connell MJ, Petroni GR et al. (1997) Adjuvant post-operative fluorouracil modulated chemotherapy combined with pelvic radiation for rectal cancer: initial results of INT 0114. Journal of Clinical Oncology 15: 2030-2039.

UKCCCR Anal Cancer Working Party (1996) Epidermoid anal cancer: Results from the UKCC-CR randomised trial of radiotherapy alone versus radiotherapy, 5-fluorouracil and mitomycin. The Lancet 348: 1049-1054.

UKCCCR Anal Cancer Working Party (2001) Trial Protocol – ACT II. The second UK Phase III Anal Cancer Trial: A trial of chemoradiation and maintenance therapy for patients with anal cancer. UKCCCR Colorectal Cancer Group.

Weinstein SM (1993) Principles and Practice of Intra-Venous Therapy, 5th edn. Lippincott.

World Health Organization (1979) WHO Handbook for Reporting Results of Cancer Treatment. WHO offset publication, No. 43. Geneva: WHO.

Young A, Rea D (2001) In: Kerr D, Young A, Hobbs R (eds) ABC of Colorectal Cancer. London: BMJ Books.

Chapter 8

Palliative nursing care

Claire Taylor

This chapter intends to impart a broad conceptualization of palliative care: one that values individuals' lives and aims to offer patients' the best quality of life possible. It addresses palliative care principles applicable to the care of patients with advanced colorectal cancer.

Case scenario 1

Jo is 76. He had surgery for a colonic cancer three years ago. He was found to have recurrence of his disease just under a year ago, when he complained of feeling 'off-colour' and losing weight. He has just been told by the hospital specialist that his last six months of chemotherapy have not shrunk the metastases found in the liver and the cancer has now spread to his lungs. On discussion it is felt that he is too unwell to undergo further chemotherapy. He appears to accept the situation and agrees that he feels too weak to manage more hospital treatment. He asks: 'So what happens to me now?'

The above scenario illustrates the difficult questions we associate with palliative care. It is hoped that this chapter answers the 'what now?', offering tangible and positive solutions to patients and their carers. Although there is good evidence how this approach can and does help, it is often viewed as a poor successor to cure-oriented approaches and may therefore be offered as a last resort when all else is perceived to have failed. It is suggested that this philosophy of care be made available much earlier in a patient's plan of care; it can then be seen as both complementary, or as an alternative to treatments directed at treating the disease. It is suitable for all patients with a life-threatening disease, including incurable colorectal cancer.

This chapter demonstrates that, in situations where providing care over cure becomes the priority, patients can still be offered hope: involvement, respect, freedom from pain, or maybe a decrease in distress. It highlights that a partnership with the patient is required to provide individualized, appropriate and supportive treatment. It discusses some of the common physical symptoms and psychological reactions experienced by patients with advanced colorectal cancer, indicating useful initial strategies for managing them.

Later in this chapter, there is a brief reference to complementary treatments, other support agencies and a description of typical community palliative care provision. First, an overview of what palliative care is and where palliative nursing fits within it.

What is palliative care?

A much quoted and illustrative definition of palliative care is: 'the active total care of patients whose disease is not responsive to curative treatment' (WHO, 1990). It illustrates that palliative care extends beyond just the support of patients with advanced disease: it actively responds to the whole person to promote holistic well-being. First and foremost, it aims to improve quality of life by controlling symptoms such as pain, through assessment and then management of any psychological, social and spiritual problems.

Optimum symptom management may involve using many different cancer treatments such as surgery, chemotherapy and radiotherapy. The key difference is that they would not be used to remove disease. They should be offered only when the benefit of such treatments can potentially outweigh any expected side effects. Such treatments can play an important role in palliation, e.g. radiotherapy to relieve bony metastatic pain. They may be useful up to the point when they may be simply prolonging the process of dying. Twycross (1995) then believes that we can best help a patient by giving death a chance.

Palliative care thus affirms life, neither hastening nor postponing the normal process of dying. It includes terminal care, which is the support required for a patient at the end of life, extending to bereavement support. The culture that prevails within not only biomedical settings, but also our society, makes death a sensitive issue. The cultural reduction in our intimacy with death has resulted in a 'death-denying society': an orientation to cure at all costs, increasing life and death boundaries (Hockey, 1990), and decreasing moral and religious conscience of death's meaning. Society's lack of contact with the dying can understandably potentiate great difficulty in dealing with it. This may be why palliative care specialists are particularly valued, and associated with, terminal care.

Palliative nursing care

Palliative nursing care involves helping the patient grow, heal, grieve or whatever he or she needs to achieve hope, comfort, peace and providing quality of life. It also presents an opportunity to work therapeutically and uniquely with each patient. It perhaps differs from a more acute approach, in making the patient central to all decisions and care provided. Individuality of care and a nurse–patient partnership are defining components. Indeed, this relationship 'together with knowledge and skills, is the essence of palliative care nursing' (Coyle, 2001). It embraces good assessment and communication skills, knowledge of the strategies to manage common symptoms and firm understandings of the principles of palliative care. 'Expressive skills' such as being with the patient, comforting, informing and sharing plans of care are essential (Wright, 1991).

Palliative care nursing includes rehabilitation skills, offering advice on the management of their lives and helping patients to achieve whatever degree of control and/or independence is possible. Nursing care should therefore enable these patients to live as fully, comfortably and enjoyably as possible, irrespective of their quantity of life. McIntyre and Cioppa (1984) suggest the following four nursing measures that may help attain this:

1. Helping patients understand actions of drugs and goals of therapies
2. Discussing rationale for treatments
3. Exploring fears and fantasies associated with the cancer experience
4. Encouraging active participation in decision-making and care.

There is a clear and independent function for the nurse who provides palliative care. After cessation of curative treatments, there may be situations when other health care professionals visibly withdraw their support, providing opportunity and freedom to work closely with the patient. Although the palliative nurse specialist must work within a team, he or she may be the best person to co-ordinate activities, and lead the patient's plan of care. Palliative care nursing also offers a strong advocacy role, supporting the patient in questioning treatment alternatives and opening up dialogue with his or her physician on the appropriateness of the care being offered. Through familiarity with the patient, the nurse can be instrumental in resolving conflicts between patient and carers and encouraging honest communication.

The patient with advanced colorectal cancer

If we consider that at least a third of colorectal cancer patients are not curable at the time of presentation, clearly there is a great need for palliative care provision within this patient group. The nurse's role in supporting patients with colorectal cancer through this time is not specifically addressed in the literature, and so reference is made to relevant research in colorectal cancer and more generic palliative care publications.

The argument for special consideration to be given to this client group, starts anatomically: 'bowels' are a taboo topic in polite society, alongside cancer and death. As one patient with advanced colorectal cancer said:

> You feel kind of embarrassed, it's a terrible disease.

Cancer in itself can be an isolating experience, but the private and potentially humiliating nature of this disease may compound communication for a colorectal cancer patient requiring palliative care. Another patient described his feelings of being very alone:

> This change in my functions is going to happen to my body and nobody else's body.

It may bring added concerns about loss of control and loss or change in normal bodily function as a result of the effect of the nature of their disease and the treatments. These experiences can create a state of personal distress, because the body image feels altered, impaired and possibly dysfunctional to the individual (Price, 1993). Limited social functioning, often through perceived stigmatization, is therefore not surprisingly evidenced in this patient group: Devlin et al. (1971) highlighted this phenomenon in patients with stomas, and MacDonald and Anderson (1985) found, five years after diagnosis, that some patients still felt disabled by their bowel function, a quarter of their sample leaving their house less often than before surgery.

Sprangers et al.'s (1993) extensive literature review confirmed the limitations in quality of life a year after surgery, in particular: bowel function, negative body image, social functioning and sexual functioning. Bliss and Johnston's (1995) study also revealed that patients with colorectal cancer had fears about socializing, normality and control. These feelings and self-imposed social restrictions can only be assumed to worsen as the disease advances and begins to affect the form and function of other bodily parts. Ascites, cachexia and lymphoedema are all very visible examples of physiological changes that may compound the distress of patients with advanced colorectal cancer.

There is little research orientated to identifying or improving the palliative care needs of colorectal cancer patients. Maguire et al.'s (1999) study of key physical complaints in the terminal phase of this disease highlighted appetite loss, pain and nausea as the main physical symptoms and found that over a third had an affective disorder. Two of the particular difficulties in palliative management of these patients are felt to be intermittent subacute intestinal obstruction and advanced/recurrent rectal cancer pain, which are mentioned under 'Treatments'.

The palliative care team

Teamwork is essential in palliative care, because no single discipline can meet all the patients' and carers' needs. There will be variation on team membership, but it will include a palliative care consultant and a palliative care specialist nurse as the minimum core team. The skills of the following professionals will also be needed: physiotherapists, occupational therapists, pharmacists, dieticians, social workers, clinical psychologists, chaplain/rabbi/priest, and other therapists. All should work towards the same goals, with co-ordination of roles and responsibilities to ensure that partnership rather than conflict occur. Teamwork should also promote continuity of care, so that the patient receives a seamless service through all care environments.

The recommendations from the Department of Health for improving outcomes in this disease (NHSE, 1997) are availability of specialist palliative care for all patients with advanced colorectal cancer. Furthermore, this provision should be accessible on a 24-hour basis. Another key recommendation states that patients should be allowed to remain in the place that they prefer, whether this be in a hospital, hospice or at home. It is known that not all patients who would like to die at home are able to do so. This may be as a result of the burden of care presently placed on carers and the inadequate community services in many areas to support them. There has recently been investment in education and support for community nurses, which will, it is hoped, improve palliative nursing care provision to patients and their carers at home.

The palliative care team's role within the colorectal cancer team involves the provision of education and advice on palliative care as well as direct patient care in managing symptoms of advanced disease. They can also offer more specialized psychological and social support to patients and their carers. Their presence at the multidisciplinary team (MDT) meetings is recommended. They bring a different perspective and add valuable insights on the values and beliefs of the patient and family that may impact on any decisions made. They may share the responsibility of a patient's management with other members of the team and use such meetings to improve interprofessional communication. The role of the palliative care team within site-specific cancer MDTs is thus increasingly being recognized.

Treatments

This section aims to present an overview of the treatments used for patients with advanced colorectal cancer and highlight that treatment decision-making can be complex, often suggesting several solutions. As discussed in Chapter 5, there are a variety of reasons for palliative surgical management, including cytoreduction, ablative procedures, symptom relief, pain control and nutritional support. The role of palliative chemotherapy and radiotherapy is discussed in Chapter 7.

Integral to treatment decision-making is patient involvement, honest and comprehensive information giving, and team management. Asking the following two questions often helps:

- 'What is the patient's priority?'
- 'What are we trying to achieve?'

Case scenario 2

Des is a fit 63-year-old man. He has previously had an anterior resection. He now presents with pain, tenesmus and altered bowel habit. He is found to have an obstructing peri-anastomotic recurrence of a rectosigmoid cancer and liver metastases. The surgeon tells him that he may benefit symptomatically from a re-resection by way of either a Hartmann's closure with a proximal colostomy or abdominoperineal excision of the rectum. He does not like the sound of the stoma, but is warned that his bowel is likely to obstruct in the next few weeks. He asks: 'What other options are there?'

This is a common scenario since recurrence at the site of the primary resection or around the anastomosis is the second most common site of recurrent colorectal cancer. Clearly any decision needs to be made on an individual basis according to the patient preference, general health and the benefit versus side effects of having major surgery. In Des's case we know that he is relatively fit now and he could be expected to recover functionally from surgery within 6–8 weeks. He would need to understand that his disease is incurable and that his survival is likely to be less than a year (Polk and Spratt, 1983), even with surgical treatment, if he wants to make a fully informed decision.

Alternatively, symptoms of bowel obstruction can be successfully managed medically using drugs such as morphine, buscopan, dexamethasone and octreotide (Frank, 1997). This option would be much worse prognostically; the mean survival for patients with malignant bowel obstruction treated non-surgically is just under two months (Gallick et al., 1985). He could also consider a combination of chemotherapy and radiotherapy to treat the recurrence in both the bowel and the liver. The radiotherapy would typically involve 25 fractions to the pelvis, with the main side effect being radiation proctitis. Chemotherapy may involve a Hickmann line, weekly trips to the hospital as an outpatient or fortnightly 2-day stays, both over a 3-month period. The side effects may be tolerable but there may be only a small and temporary symptomatic improvement, and this would be unlikely to prevent obstruction and improve survival (Hoskin and Makin, 1998).

Colonic stenting is an endoscopic approach proving to be a feasible, effective adjunct and alternative to surgery for managing large bowel obstruction. It provides lasting and successful palliation, with minimal morbidity and no mortality associated with the procedure (Arnell et al., 1998). Baron et al. (1998) reported that stent placement was technically possible in 94 per cent of their sample of patients with palliative disease, and 82 per cent achieved relief from obstruction.

Another option would be a much simpler operation to create a proximal diverting colostomy with postoperative pelvic radiotherapy, particularly if there is more extensive pelvic disease, which may offer better palliation of his pain and tenesmus discomfort for several months (Gunderson et al., 1980). So although the surgery might at face value seem the best option, if he felt adamant that he did not want a stoma this would clearly not be the best decision for him. After making that decision, it is likely that he would need to consider the other options with the oncologist, palliative care team and his family.

The nursing role would first involve current symptom management, possibly using oral and topical morphine, stool softeners and a non-prokinetic antiemetic such as cyclizine if he felt nauseous. Other drugs such as a topical anti-inflammatory or anaesthetic, amitriptyline and nifedipine may be required, depending on the description of the rectal pain. Second, it may be valuable, after and between consultations, to offer to listen, explain and summarize the situation. Feeling that his aspirations are respected and that ultimately his decision will be supported is an important nursing function. Sometimes a patient's decision may conflict with the personal beliefs of the nurse, e.g. if he decided he wanted survival, at the expense of all else, it can be difficult to remain non-judgemental.

Liver therapies

The most common focus of recurrent colorectal cancer is the liver. There is now a small possibility of cure for patients with liver metastases through surgical resection of a section of the liver. Careful staging is required to assess size, amount and position of liver disease, and to confirm that there is no extrahepatic disease. In general, the criteria are: less than three metastases in not more than one lobe, no larger than 5 cm in diameter, although the 'curative' indications are evolving. Other treatments for liver metastases are available that target the cancer directly, causing minimal collateral damage: cryotherapy, thermal ablation and hepatic laser therapy.

Nursing management of physical symptoms

Three common symptoms experienced by patients with colorectal cancer requiring palliative care nursing are described in this section: pain, anorexia/cachexia syndrome and constipation. The average patient with advanced malignant disease will, however, experience up to seven different symptoms at any one time. Thus, when caring for these patients, it is likely that more than one symptom will require active attention. This requires a detailed assessment of each symptom's history, nature, pattern and frequency, alongside eliciting measures that alleviate and exacerbate. It is important that the cause of each symptom is elicited, and not just assumed to be caused by advancing disease.

Pain

Pain is perhaps the most feared and most prominent of symptoms experienced by patients, even though a quarter of cancer patients never experience it (Twycross, 1997). Physical pain impairs functioning in social, spiritual and psychological health and, in turn, is exacerbated by suffering in these dimensions. Pain charts can assist in assessing the severity of the pain, e.g. using a visual analogue scale and/or body maps to highlight sites of pain. Fewer than 30 per cent of patients have just one site of pain (Grond, 1996). When assessing pain it must be viewed as a multifactorial symptom. The pain will have its own meaning to the patient: it may signal increasing disability, dependence and decreasing life; therefore these need exploration. Patients should be told that pain is not inevitable, painkillers are not addictive or an acquiescent step, and that they have a right to adequate pain relief.

Cases where the affective component outweighs the cognitive one indicate the importance of supportive and holistic measures alongside pharmacological ones. Alternatives to analgesics include counselling, relaxation, modifications to way of life, heat pads, transcutaneous electrical nerve stimulation (TENS), cancer treatments including hormone therapy and nerve blocks. Once an initial treatment regimen is agreed, it must be reviewed regularly to ensure that the most effective treatment response is maintained. In the inpatient setting, this means daily, possibly even more frequently, depending on the severity and distress of the symptom.

It is important to involve the patient in the discussion about treatment; gaining trust and co-operation improves compliance and confidence. Goals can be set with their aspirations in focus, e.g. free of pain at night, free of pain when reading and, ultimately, free of pain when washing and dressing. These need to be viewed and achieved incrementally, rather than letting the patient assume that a new regimen will work tomorrow. If a patient is very anxious, it may take up to four weeks to achieve maximum pain relief (Twycross, 1997). There are some key points to remember when using analgesic drugs in cancer pain, well cited elsewhere:

- Analgesics should be given 'by mouth, by the clock and by the ladder'.
- The strength should be titrated up accordingly, using the analgesic ladder (Figure 8.1).
- Morphine remains the drug of first choice in severe pain.
- Fears of respiratory depression and psychological dependence are unfounded in this setting when the dose is titrated up the ladder accordingly.
- Until the analgesic requirements are known, patients should stay on quick release formulations. If conversion to slow-release medications is made, breakthrough quick-release analgesia should always be available as needed.

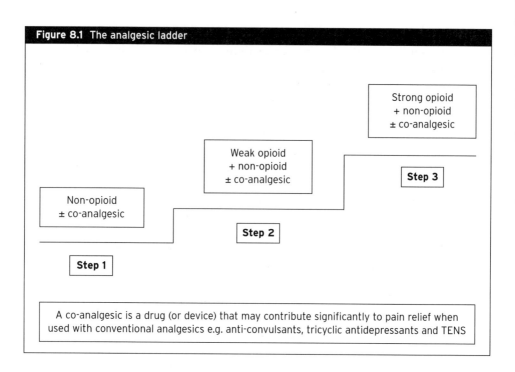

Figure 8.1 The analgesic ladder

Strong opioid
+ non-opioid
± co-analgesic

Weak opioid
+ non-opioid
± co-analgesic

Step 3

Non-opioid
± co-analgesic

Step 2

Step 1

A co-analgesic is a drug (or device) that may contribute significantly to pain relief when used with conventional analgesics e.g. anti-convulsants, tricyclic antidepressants and TENS

Anorexia and weight loss

These can be coupled together as the anorexia/cachexia syndrome, associated with involuntary weight loss and progressive wasting. The patient may also experience early satiety, nausea, fatigue, anaemia and change in body image (Bruera, 1998). It is one of the most common symptoms in advanced malignancy and is associated with poorer outcomes and compromised quality of life. Weisman and Worden's (1977) analysis that colorectal cancer patients had low levels of psychosocial concerns in comparison with the other cancer patients, has not been supported in other studies, in particular Maguire et al.'s study (1999).

Schag et al.'s study (1992) noted the salience of functional status in colorectal cancer patients postoperatively: problems with energy and weight loss often persist and cause significant rehabilitation problems. Both the body's inflammatory response to the cancer and tumour byproducts create metabolic abnormalities that cause protein loss, anorexia and increased fat metabolism.

The management of anorexia and weight loss requires attention to the complex physiological, behavioural and psychological variables that interplay in causation. Exclusion of reversible causes such as anxiety, nausea and poor oral health, and referral to a dietician are good initial strategies. Pharmacological interventions include three groups of drugs: pro-kinetic agents, e.g. metoclopramide, corticosteroids e.g. dexamethasone 2–4 mg/day on a 1-week trial, and a progesterone, e.g. megestrol acetate, to stimulate appetite. Important nursing measures are assessment, explanation and teaching subjects such as how to improve food intake, maintenance of good oral hygiene and management of fatigue. These symptoms can create great frustration and distress. Pleasure associated with food disappears, mealtimes become stressful, and carers experience guilt or failure if they can't produce the 'right' food.

Constipation

Of the range of bowel problems that can be experienced in this patient group, constipation is a symptom affecting at least half the patients with advanced malignant disease. In defining constipation, difficulty in defecation is more important than infrequency of stools. Although the aetiology is multifactorial, patients on opioid analgesia are at greater risk and need to take laxatives. However, when assessing cause, opioids often get blamed when immobility, impaired fluid and food intake, and disease-impairing bowel motility may be equally causative.

The treatment of constipation is highlighted as:

- Treat cause if possible, e.g. encourage mobilization, increase oral fluids and modify drug regimen.
- Use laxatives – titrate dose to achieve ease of defecation.

Note that a combination of softening and stimulant drugs produces the best results with fewer adverse effects and smaller medicine volumes (Sykes, 1997).

Psychological support

This section briefly covers the following five areas: communication, information, anger, denial and fear. The distress of a patient with advanced colorectal cancer may well be compounded by many different reactions: fear, anger, and denial have been selected as three that are commonly encountered.

Attending and listening are two of the most fundamental communication skills (Morrison and Burnard, 1997). Even if there is no more than 2 minutes to spend with a patient, a deliberate focus on the person needing help can be enough to hear how he or she is feeling. At a deeper level this can extend to hearing the patient's 'overall' message through attention to non-verbal communication and transmission of a feeling of empathy or resonance, as the nurse begins to see the world from the patient's perspective. Radwin's (2000) study of oncology patients' perceptions of quality nursing care found that a comprehensive knowledge base needed to be coupled with certain psychosocial attributes – care, partnership, rapport and an individualized approach – to be perceived as excellent care.

The four main sources of dissatisfaction with health care professionals' communication skills among persons with life-threatening illness are (McSkimming et al., 1999):

1. Too much focus on medical and physical interventions
2. Insufficient information
3. Apparent discomfort in talking about death
4. Not including family members in the conversation.

The importance of information in helping patients understand their illness experiences, in regulating the emotional effects of the diagnosis, and preparing them for adjustments to their life is clear. People with advanced colorectal cancer need to be offered information about how to ameliorate or manage the consequences of their disease, as well as what to expect and how to manage any potential problems, in order to feel empowered and independent. A proactive approach in information-giving is advised.

In consideration of the particular psychological support needed by these patients, naturally any generalizations should be treated with caution. Colorectal cancer patients have expressed dissatisfaction with health care professionals' management of some of their physical and functional problems after treatment (Sprangers et al., 1993). In Knowles et al.'s study (1999), patients with colorectal cancer had high information needs at points through their chemotherapy treatment, half the patients perceiving a lack of treatment information, despite availability of specialist oncology knowledge. Inevitably all patients with advancing colorectal disease and/or anticipating of death will have some informational needs and responses or concerns that need acknowledgment.

Anger

Dealing with anger can be difficult: its cause is often misinterpreted, and it may elicit personal feelings of defensiveness or hurt. The first step in its management is considering why someone is showing anger, looking beyond the obvious or stated reasons. Sometimes there will be a reasonable and justified cause for complaint within their treatment experiences, which will need to be resolved.

A common reason for anger is essentially a perception of injustice in having this disease: the way the disease makes them feel, the loss of control and/or powerlessness over outcome. The key initially is not to assume understanding, but instead to let feelings be heard. Hopefully acknowledging the anger, encouraging calm and controlled discussion, and addressing all the reasons why they feel angry will move the patient forward. They may then become quite sad or fearful. Sometimes they may not be ready to let go of their anger and gaining recognition that this is their coping mechanism, by reviewing how they have coped previously, may be as much as is achievable. If anger persists, consideration should also be given to whether this is part of another condition, such as depression, that requires specialist help.

Denial

Case scenario 3

Enid was admitted to hospital complaining of extreme weakness and frequent bloody diarrhoea. She had lost two stone over several months, had no appetite and was anaemic. On being told she had a growth in her bowel, she refused further tests and treatment. The palliative care team's approach was initially to gain her trust then elicit what she understood, assess current symptoms and understand her wishes for the future. She had suspected something serious, knew her body was very poorly, but did not want to know any more than this. Her priority was managing the diarrhoea and her sore mouth so that she could enjoy food again. Tranexamic acid was commenced orally to try to reduce bleeding in the bowel, plus loperamide as needed until the diarrhoea became manageable. Her mouth required an anaesthetic mouthwash to be used before meals, an antifungal mouthwash after meals and regular sips of fluid to aid mastication. She wanted to stay in bed and thus required use of the commode. Her wishes alongside advice on good mouth and perianal care were discussed with the nursing team.

Faced with difficult news, most people will respond with denial or acceptance. In this scenario, Enid displayed some degree of denial and wanted practical help, oriented in the present with no discussion of more sensitive issues. Working on her terms allowed her main concerns to be addressed and an improved quality of life to be achieved. Glaser and Strauss (1976) found that patients used some typical denying strategies, including significantly extending their own prognosis, orientation to the future over the present, positively comparing themselves to others, becoming intensively active and blocking communication. Some patients may start using denial when they approach death and may die without acknowledging that they are dying. This may be a helpful coping mechanism. Challenging denial when it serves to decrease a patient's distress may be dangerous. Rather, it may be a case for examining personal or others' feelings and expectations of what constitutes coping and 'a good death'.

A scenario of mutual pretence can develop, when day-to-day activities mask what is really happening and limit honest dialogue. This often creates tension between carers and patient, limits service provision, and may prevent completion of unfinished business before death (Rando, 1986). Only when a patient is not coping with feelings is it advisable to redress them (Regnard and Tempest, 1998). It is helpful to assess whether the patient's level of denial is consistent through the day, or if at any time – often in the early hours of the morning – the patient feels any different. If the latter is the case, there is opportunity to work with these feelings and gently challenge any inconsistencies in their accounts. A change in awareness may take time, and continued support is required.

Fear

Few people do not have some fears of the dying process. It is commonly believed that death from cancer will be a painful, undignified and uncontrollable process. Patients often worry about dependence on or causing suffering to others and may also feel afraid of an uncertain ending. Many fears may be irrational and overwhelming until shared. It is not possible to give absolutes or always be truly accurate about expected symptoms, treatment responses or timescales. However, patients with advanced colorectal cancer who do have time to accept that they are dying are unlikely to have a sudden and traumatic death. Many patients die gradually, becoming increasingly fatigued and sleepy and decreasingly hungry, active and aware of their environment before death.

Families will also undergo stages of psychological adjustment and can be expected to experience similar emotions of grief. (For literature on grief reactions, refer to Kübler-Ross (1969) and Parkes (1986).) As carers, they may need time to discuss their feelings alongside practical advice on how to care for someone dying, signs suggesting imminent death, and what to do after death has occurred. Talking through the possible scenarios, the dying process and what support will be available will help them prepare, plan, and feel more confident in their responsibilities. This fittingly leads us on to spiritual care.

Spiritual support

Raimal was a 56-year-old woman who had been diagnosed with an inoperable locally advanced sigmoid cancer. She was referred to the district nurse and community Macmillan nurse at the time of diagnosis, to manage her constipation and pain. After a couple of visits they established an effective and tolerable regimen of analgesics and laxatives. However, she still felt awful: she felt weak, had pain all over her tummy and could not sleep. She was a quiet woman, who was reluctant to express how she felt. She liked to leave her family to make her decisions and offered no ideas on how we could make her feel better. It became apparent through spending time with her that she had significant spiritual distress. Assessing all the reasons why she couldn't sleep at night was the opening to understanding this: she saw the family's distress, could not 'make it better' and felt 'useless'. Most importantly she would not be able to arrange her son's marriage. She also felt she had insufficient time to accept her prognosis and that she was destined to endure a suffering that she could not face.

A person facing death (which may be when they first hear that they have cancer) often engages in a personal spiritual journey. They may question what life and death mean, what their life has meant, what is important to them and what their fears and hopes of death are. People generally need support to help them work through such profound thoughts. As nurses, we are in an ideal position to help patients overcome spiritual pain. We should aim for three goals in spiritual care (Highfield, 1992):

1. Self-acceptance
2. Achievement of a sense of meaning and purpose in life
3. Achievement of a relationship with other/supreme other, characterized by love, trust, forgiveness and hope.

In the scenario above, the woman's description of pain and her regular reference to suffering were good indicators of her spiritual distress. However, it took considerable time and gentle but persistent probing for her to reveal her most significant problem. Once she felt safe to share her thoughts, she did actually talk at length and it was clear that skilled facilitation of dialogue between her and her family was the next step in helping her. In many cases, it may be enough to listen as patients talk through their life and, in doing so, search for meaning within it. If life is valued and seen as meaningful, having to confront this being taken from them naturally provokes a sense of loss. This is often referred to as anticipatory grief.

It is felt that spiritual support is the dimension most likely to be neglected within holistic assessment, with misconceptions of religion's role within it. Although a person's religious beliefs are likely to have significant impact on such thoughts and values, spirituality has wider existential associations. When assessing spiritual needs, it may be useful to categorize spirituality into three components (Kaye, 1990):

1. The past: any sense of regret, guilt or failure or any memories that remain painful, that they feel able to share.
2. The present: how do they see life right now - how are they accepting their diagnosis and prognosis, do they feel it is unfair, do they feel angry, sad and do they feel supported?
3. The future: fears, degree of hope.

When time is limited, exploring these components may feel ambitious and unachievable. However, even doing ordinary things for people such as assisting with personal grooming, helping them see beauty about themselves or, for example, arranging for grandchildren to visit, can all help patients to find sense and value in their life. There may also be somebody better placed to hear the more difficult questions such as: 'Why me?', 'Why has God let this happen?' and 'How will I die?' While not every question needs an answer, sometimes a referral to a chaplain or psychologist may be beneficial to provide skilled discussion, and opportunity for prayer, reading and reflection. Recognition of when a referral to another agency is necessary is an important nursing skill.

In summary, multidimensional assessment of each presenting symptom is required. No meaningful conversation can take place unless the uppermost symptoms that the patient is experiencing are first alleviated (Marks, 1988). Hence a patient who is so distracted with anxiety may well need anxiolytics and relaxation therapy before counselling can begin.

Social support

Social support is critical to individuals coping with such a major life event as the diagnosis of cancer (Ell et al., 1989; Lackner et al., 1994). It is known that higher levels of support result in better adjustment to this disease (Ell et al., 1988). It may be even more important, in this disease, when its effects are known to be socially restricting or stigmatizing. Social support should redress this sense of isolation. The patient's main support system is likely to be his or her family and friends. Spouses of patients with colorectal cancer have reported a general lack of support, because their needs get overlooked in the patient's favour (Oberst and James, 1988). They too will be feeling the impact of the patient's disease and treatment. They may feel stressed and exhausted but are expected to continue to cope and respond positively (Dunkel-Schetter, 1984). These key people will feel more able to provide help and support to the patient if they also feel involved, informed and supported.

Outside the family and friend network, support is available from health care professionals such as Macmillan nurses, who specialize in offering support to patients with cancer. This support aims to facilitate the adjustment of the individual and his or her family to the diagnosis and its effects. Macmillan nurses are often involved from the time of diagnosis and will take referrals from patients and/or relatives. In the community, specialist palliative care nurses and Macmillan nurses may be collectively referred to as 'home care'. They may take referrals based on severity of patient symptoms, adequacy of existing support structures and prognosis of the patient, for instance; some stipulate a prognosis of less than six months. They work with the patient's carers and particularly through the district nurse to offer specialist knowledge in symptom management, support and to co-ordinate the patient's care.

They may transfer a patient to the local specialist inpatient unit if the carer needs a rest/respite, if carers feel unable to support the patient's death at home or, more usually, if the patient has symptoms and/or complex needs that cannot be relieved in their present setting. Sometimes a referral to specialist palliative day care, often simply referred to as 'day care', is enough to give the carer a break one day a week, and the patient the opportunity to feel pampered, or perhaps just to forget their cancer as they engage in activities happening around them. It is a service 'which enhances the independence and quality of life of patients through rehabilitation, physiotherapy and occupational therapy, the management of symptoms and the provision of psychological and social support' (DoH, 1999).

Most organizations for people with cancer provide support for close family and friends, e.g. CancerBACUP and Macmillan Cancer Relief. There are now a few charities that are solely oriented to patients diagnosed with colorectal cancer, but they do not provide a specific palliative care resource. Local branches of national organizations often exist, aimed at providing on-going personalized support that may provide patients with the confidence and direction that they need (Evans, 1995), e.g. the British Colostomy/Ileostomy Association. The Red Cross is another useful organization for loan of equipment for patients being cared for at home, e.g. commodes, back boards. Often the patient's local area will have visiting or befriending schemes to offer support at home, particularly to people living alone. There may also be local bereavement support groups in addition to bereavement support offered by a palliative care team/hospice.

Complementary therapies

Complementary therapies are increasingly being used within palliative care. They may be offered within oncology centres and specialist palliative care units to complement and enhance other therapeutic interventions, or they may be employed privately by the patient. Acupuncture is perhaps one of the most accepted complementary therapies, considered by palliative care specialists to be an important technique to have available to their patients. It is used primarily to treat cancer pain, but may also be a valuable treatment for symptoms such as nausea and vomiting, respiratory problems, dry mouth and stress reduction. However, there is a lack of evidence to support its effectiveness and it has several contraindications for use within palliative care, e.g. neutropenia, altered skin sensation after radiotherapy, and steroid therapy. Two well-conducted studies on the benefits of using aromatherapy massage for cancer patients have found reductions in anxiety, and improvements in symptom control and in quality of life (Kite et al., 1998; Wilkinson et al., 1999).

Managing self

In providing palliative care we often face complex and emotionally distressing situations, affronting moral and ethical values and requiring considerable demands 'of self'. For this reason, a section on care of self has been included. Corner and Wilson-Barnett (1992) revealed nurses' vulnerabilities in providing psychological care, identifying deep and unresolved fears about their own mortality. Clearly a nurse's beliefs and attitudes to death affect the nurse–patient relationship at this time. It is necessary to acknowledge these beliefs and to accept that death is a part of life. One also needs to recognize the effect of 'self', as well as effects *on* self in such encounters. Working within this speciality carries the potential for stress and emotional exhaustion or 'burn-out'.

Copp and Dunn's (1993) interviews with nurses caring for dying patients across three settings found that the most difficult aspect of care was helping patients experiencing difficulties in adjusting to their terminal status and separation from families. Inevitably the close interpersonal relationships that nurses develop may lead to personal grief reactions when there is realization of deterioration or loss, in a patient and/or carer. Support is needed to enhance the nurse's maintenance of his or her professional boundaries (Frogatt, 1995). This will allow identification of over-involvement with patients in a way that is not beneficial to either patient or self. This support may come in the form of clinical supervision, peers, senior management and interests outside work. Any mechanism such as clinical supervision, which offers opportunity to reflect and develop self-awareness, is encouraged.

Conclusion

In this millennium our patients will, and should, expect palliative care that 'supports and not obstructs, living fully until death' (Super, 2001, p. 27). The ability of the nurse to recognize the physical, psychological, social and spiritual needs of patients with incurable disease, and to make the appropriate interventions and referrals, remain essential to the provision of good palliative care practice. Through valuing the partnership of nurses both with patients and within healthcare, the pluralistic, multidimensional challenges and barriers that face patients today can be overcome. The recent recognition of the central role that nursing plays within the colorectal multidisciplinary team offers nurses new opportunities to lead patients' care, to participate in research and to communicate more effectively with one another. The value of palliative care nursing in providing individualized, holistic and continuous care will, it is hoped, then become increasingly evident.

Government publications, evidence-based guidelines and subsequent policy changes in palliative care should continue with the same priority. These should be juxtaposed with the knowledge that guidelines inform practice, but never take precedence over individual patient wishes. Nursing patients with colorectal cancer who need palliative care is thus a challenging and paradoxical speciality, but nevertheless a rewarding one. It offers hope that something can be done, and in doing so solicits not only what skills, knowledge and experience one brings as a nurse, but what one brings as a person. Thus, in answer to Jo's question, in Scenario 1, palliative care and palliative nursing should offer the following:

- Involvement of the patient and their family
- A respect for the individual's wishes and needs of the patient and family
- A holistic approach to care
- The maintenance or improvement of quality of life (as defined by the patient)
- A multiprofessional approach to care provision.

References

Arnell T, Stamos MJ, Takahashi P, Ojha S, Sze G, Eysselein V (1998) Colonic stents in colorectal obstruction. American Surgery 64: 986-988.

Baron TH, Dean PA, Yates MR, 3rd, Canon C, Koehler RE (1998) Expandable metal stents for the treatment of colonic obstruction: techniques and outcomes. Gastroscopy and Endoscopy 47: 277-286.

Bliss J, Johnston B (1995) After diagnosis of cancer: the patient's view of life. International Journal of Palliative Nursing 1: 126-133.

Bruera E (1998) Pharmacological treatment of cachexia: any progress? Support Care Cancer 6: 109-113.

Corner J, Wilson-Barnett J (1992) The newly registered nurse and the cancer patient: An educational evaluation. International Journal of Nursing Studies 29: 177-190.

Copp G, Dunn V (1993) Frequent and difficult problems perceived by nurses caring for the dying in community, hospice and acute care settings. Palliative Medicine 7: 19-25.

Coyle N. (2001) Introduction to palliative care nursing. In: Ferrell BR, Coyle N (eds), Textbook of Palliative Nursing. Oxford: Oxford University Press.

Department of Health (1999) Palliative Care: Assessor's Checklist (Prepared by the DoH for the New Opportunities Fund in association with the National Council for Hospice and Specialist Palliative Care Service and the Hospice Information Service). London: NHS Executive, DoH.

Devlin BH, Plant JA, Griffin M (1971) Aftermath of surgery for anorectal cancer. British Medical Journal 3: 415-418.

Dunkel-Schetter C (1984) Social support and cancer: Findings based on patient interviews and their implications. Journal of Social Issues 40: 77-98.

Ell K, Nishimoto RH, Mantell J, Hamovitch M (1988) Longitudinal analysis of psychological adaptation among family members with cancer. Journal of Psychosomatic Research 32: 429-438.

Ell K, Mantell J, Hamovitch M, Nishimoto RH (1989) Social Support, Sense of Control and Coping Among Patients with Breast, Lung or Colorectal Cancer. Journal of Psychosocial Oncology 7: 63-89.

Evans BD (1995) The experiences and needs of patients attending a cancer support group. International Journal of Palliative Care 1(4): 189-194.

Frank C (1997) Medical management of intestinal obstruction in terminal care. Canadian Family Physician 43: 259-265.

Frogatt K (1995) Nurses and involvement in palliative care work. In: Richardson A, Wilson-Barnett J (eds), Nursing Research in Cancer Care. London: Scutari Press, pp. 151-164.

Gallick HL, Weaver DW et al. (1986) Intestinal obstruction in cancer patients: an assessment of risk factors and outcome. American Surgeon 52: 434-437.

Glaser BG, Strass L (1976) Awareness of Dying. New York: Aldine Publishing Co.

Grond S (1996) Assessment of cancer pain: a prospective evaluation on 2266 cancer patients referred to a pain service. Pain 64: 107-114.

Gunderson LL, Cohen AM, Welch CE (1980) Residual, inoperable or recurrent colorectal cancer: Interaction of surgery and radiotherapy. American Journal of Surgery 139: 518-525.

Highfield MF (1992) Spiritual health of oncology patients: nurses and patients perspectives. Cancer Nursing 15(1): 1-8.

Hockey J (1990) Experiences of Death. Edinburgh: Edinburgh University Press.

Hoskin P, Makin W (1998) Oncology for Palliative Medicine. Oxford: Oxford University Press.

Kaye P (1990) Symptom Control in Hospice and Palliative Care. London: Hospital Education Institution.

Kite SM, Maher EJ, Anderson K et al. (1998) Development of an aromatherapy service at a cancer centre. Palliative Medicine 12: 171-180.

Knowles G, Tierney A et al. (1999) The perceived information needs of patients receiving adjuvant chemotherapy for surgically resected colorectal cancer. European Journal of Oncology Nursing 3: 208-220.

Kübler-Ross E (1969) On Death and Dying. Englewood Cliffs, NJ: Prentice Hall Inc.

Lackner S, Goldenberg S, Arizza G, Tjoswold I (1994) The contingency of social support. Qualitative Health Research 4: 224-243.

MacDonald LD, Anderson HR (1985) The health of rectal cancer patients in the community European Journal of Surgical Oncology 11: 235-241.

McIntire SN, Cioppa AL (1984) Cancer Nursing: A developmental approach. New York: John Wiley & Sons Inc.

McSkimming S, Hodges M, Super A et al. (1999) The experience of life-threatening illness: patients and their loved ones perspectives. Journal of Palliative Medicine 2: 173-183.

Marks M (1988) Death, dying, bereavement and loss. In: Webb P (ed.), Oncology for Nurses and Health Care Professionals, 2nd edn, Vol. 2: Care and Support. London: Harper & Row, pp. 226-244.

Maguire P, Walsh S, Jeacock J, Kingston R (1999) Physical and psychological needs of patients dying from colo-rectal cancer. Palliative Medicine 13(1): 45-50.

Morrison P, Burnard P (1997) Caring and Communicating, 2nd edn. London: Macmillan Press Ltd.

National Health Service Executive (1997) Guidance on Commissioning Cancer Services: Improving Outcomes in Colorectal Cancer. London: NHSE, DoH.

Oberst MT, James RH (1988) Going Home: patients and spouse adjustment following cancer surgery. Topics in Clinical Nursing 7: 46-57.

Parkes CM (1986) Bereavement: Studies of grief in adult life, 2nd edn. London: Pelican.

Polk HC, Spratt JS (1983) Recurrent cancer of the colon. Surgical Clinics of North America 63: 151-160.

Price B (1993) Profiling the high risk altered body image patient. Senior Nurse 13(4): 17-21.

Radwin L (2000) Oncology patients' perceptions of quality nursing care. Research in Nursing and Health 23(3): 79-90.

Rando TA (1986) Loss and Anticipatory Grief. Lexington, Mass: Lexington Books.

Regnard CFB, Tempest S (1998) A Guide to Symptom Relief in Advanced Disease, 4th edn. London: Hochland & Hochland Ltd.

Schag CAC, Ganz PA et al. (1992) Quality of life in adult survivors of lung, colon and prostate cancer. Quality of Life Research 3: 127-141.

Schag TB, Gray RE, Fitch M (2000) A qualitative study of patient perspectives on colorectal cancer. Cancer Practice 8(1): 38-44.

Sprangers MAG, Te Velde A, Aaronson NK, Taal BG (1993) Quality of life following surgery for colorectal cancer: A literature review. Psycho-Oncology 2: 247-259.

Sykes NP (1997) A volunteer model for the comparison of laxatives in opioid-induced constipation. Journal of Pain and Symptom Management 11: 363-369.

Super A (2001) The context of palliative care in progressive illness. In: Ferrell BR, Coyle N (eds), Textbook of Palliative Nursing. Oxford: Oxford University Press, pp. 27-36.

Twycross R (1995) Symptom Management in Advanced Cancer. Oxford: Radcliffe Medical Press.

Twycross R (1997) Introducing Palliative Care, 2nd edn. Oxford: Radcliffe Medical Press.

Weisman AD, Worden JW (1976) The existential plight in cancer: significance of the first 100 days. International Journal of Psychiatry in Medicine 7: 1-14.

Wilkinson S, Aldridge J, Salmon I, Cain E, Wilson B (1999) An evaluation of aromatherapy massage in palliative care. Palliative Medicine 13: 409-417.

World Health Organization (1990) Cancer Pain Relief and Palliative Care. Report of WHO Expert Committee. WHO Technical Report Series, 804. Geneva; WHO.

Wright S (1991) Facilitating therapeutic nursing and independent practice. In: McMahon R, Pearson A (eds), Nursing as Therapy. London: Chapman & Hall, pp. 102-119.

Index

Page numbers in *italics* refer to tables or figures